MANUAL OF NUCLEAR MEDICINE PROCEDURES

MANUAL OF
NUCLEAR MEDICINE PROCEDURES

Raman Mistry

Principal Medical Physics Technician
Department of Nuclear Medicine
Guy's Hospital
London

SPRINGER-SCIENCE+BUSINESS MEDIA, B.V.

© 1988 Raman Mistry

Originally published by Chapman and Hall in 1988

Typeset in 10/12pt Optima by Photoprint,
Torquay, Devon

ISBN 978-0-412-30240-4

British Library Cataloguing in Publication Data

Mistry, Raman
    Manual of nuclear medicine procedures.
    1. Man. Diagnosis. Radiography. Use of
    radioisotope scanning. Techniques
    I. Title
    616.07′575

ISBN 978-0-412-30240-4   ISBN 978-1-4899-3134-4 (eBook)
DOI 10.1007/978-1-4899-3134-4

To my wife, Kamu,
for her love and support
and my children, Kamini and Bhavin

CONTENTS

PREFACE   xi

FOREWORD by Professor M. N. Maisey   xiii

ABBREVIATIONS   xv

PARTIAL LIST OF RADIONUCLIDES
USABLE WITH GAMMA CAMERAS   xvii

1 RENAL IMAGING STUDIES   1
   1.1 Radiopharmaceuticals   2
   1.2 Standard dynamic two-kidney renal study using
        $^{99}Tc^m$-DPTA   4
   1.3 Two-kidney renal study using frusemide diuresis   8
   1.4 Ureteric reflux study   12
   1.5 Residual bladder volume estimation   14
   1.6 Two-kidney renal study using ^{123}I-hippuran   16
   1.7 Renal transplant study   19
   1.8 Static renal study using $^{99}Tc^m$-DMSA   23

2 GLOMERULAR FILTRATION RATE   27
   2.1 Dilution and dispensing of ^{51}Cr-EDTA   28
   2.2 Technique of GFR estimation using ^{51}Cr-EDTA   31

3 BONE IMAGING STUDIES   35
   3.1 Radiopharmaceuticals   36
   3.2 Routine bone imaging   37
   3.3 Routine bone imaging using a *scanning* gamma camera   40
   3.4 Bone flow study   42
   3.5 Sacroiliac quantitation study   44

4 LIVER–SPLEEN STUDIES   45
   4.1 Radiopharmaceuticals   46
   4.2 Liver–spleen imaging   48
   4.3 Bone marrow imaging   50
   4.4 Spleen imaging with denatured RBCs   52

    4.5 Splenic clearance study   54
    4.6 Peritoneal (LeVeen) shunt study   56

5 GASTRIC STUDIES   58
    5.1 Radiopharmaceuticals   60
    5.2 Hepatobiliary imaging   64
    5.3 Gastric (oesophageal) reflux   66
    5.4 Gastric emptying (dual label)   68
    5.5 Biliary (duodenogastric) reflux   70
    5.6 Oesophageal clearance   74
    5.7 Meckel's diverticulum imaging   76
    5.8 Localization of gastrointestinal bleeding with $^{99}Tc^{m}$-RBC   78
    5.9 Salivary gland imaging (static)   80
    5.10 Salivary gland imaging (dynamic)   82

6 LUNG IMAGING STUDIES   86
    6.1 Radiopharmaceuticals   88
    6.2 Perfusion lung imaging   90
    6.3 $^{81}Kr^{m}$ ventilation lung imaging   92
    6.4 $^{99}Tc^{m}$-DTPA aerosol ventilation lung imaging   94
    6.5 Ventilation lung imaging using ^{133}Xe 96

7 CARDIAC STUDIES   98
    7.1 Radiopharmaceuticals   100
    7.2 Stress testing   104
    7.3 ^{201}Tl myocardial imaging   108
    7.4 Infarct imaging   110
    7.5 Gated red-cell studies   112
    7.6 First-pass study for left-to-right shunt detection   118
    7.7 MAA blood flow study for right-to-left shunt detection   122

8 NEUROLOGICAL STUDIES   125
    8.1 Radiopharmaceuticals   126
    8.2 Cerebral flow study   128
    8.3 Static brain imaging   130
    8.4 Cisternography   132
    8.5 Ventriculoatrial and ventriculoperitoneal shunts   134

9 ENDOCRINE STUDIES   136
    9.1 Radiopharmaceuticals   138
    9.2 $^{99}Tc^{m}$ thyroid imaging and uptake   141
    9.3 ^{123}I thyroid imaging and uptake   144
    9.4 ^{123}I-perchlorate discharge test   146
    9.5 ^{131}I whole-body imaging   148
    9.6 Parathyroid imaging   151

9.7   Adrenal cortex imaging   156
9.8 ^{131}I-MIBG phaeochromocytoma imaging   158
9.9   Testicular imaging   160
9.10   TRH test   162
9.11   Calcitonin provocation test   163

10 HAEMATOLOGY STUDIES   164
10.1   Radiopharmaceuticals   166
10.2   Red-cell mass estimation   168
10.3   Red-cell survival and sequestration studies   170
10.4 ^{51}Cr gastrointestinal blood loss study   176
10.5   Plasma volume estimation using ^{125}I-HSA   178
10.6 ^{111}In leucocyte imaging study   180

11 MISCELLANEOUS STUDIES   183
11.1   Radiopharmaceuticals   184
11.2 ^{67}Ga imaging   185
11.3   Lacrimal scintigraphic imaging   188
11.4   Gastrointestinal protein loss estimation using
        ^{51}Cr-chromic chloride   190
11.5   Lymphatic imaging   192

INDEX   195

PREFACE

This manual is designed primarily to be of assistance to trainee nuclear medicine technicians and radiographers. It will also be of value to those who are already trained in the safe handling and use of radionuclides for imaging, as a rapid reference for routine and non-routine nuclear medicine imaging procedures.

The procedures described were largely developed or modified at the Nuclear Medicine Department, Guy's Hospital, London, with regular updates during the last 10 years.

The main body of each chapter deals with the technical aspects of radionuclide imaging and each chapter contains a section on the preparation procedure for the relevant radiopharmaceuticals used with brief summaries of the aim of any data analyses using a computer system.

Although the methods described do not represent the only way to carry out such procedures, they have all been evaluated extensively and are known to give satisfactory results.

I would like to record my thanks to all members of this department who have helped by providing advice, comments and data. In particular, I would like to thank Dr Colin Lazarus for his help with the radiopharmaceuticals sections. I am most grateful to Dr Sue Clarke and Dr Ignac Fogelman for checking the manuscripts and finally to Professor Michael Maisey without whose constant encouragement and support this work would not have been possible.

FOREWORD

The development of nuclear medicine was initially a slow process. It was only with the introduction of imaging – initially rectilinear scanners and, later, gamma cameras – and the discovery of Technetium 99m, that the subject assumed an identity of its own and became a recognized medical speciality.

This manual evolved from a series of internal worksheets which formed the basis of the departmental procedure manual, and it fills a gap in the available literature and should go a long way in standardizing the discipline. It is the integration of years of careful analysis, rejection and improvement, and provides full details of reliable methods which have been tried and tested, and developed and refined over the years.

Nuclear medicine, as with many applications of science to medicine, stands or falls on technical quality – the ability of everyone involved in the procedure consistently to produce data and images of the highest quality achievable; without this, diagnosis is at best unreliable, and at worst may become critically dangerous to the patient. The theoretical basis of a test using radio-isotopes may be sound and the skill of the physician interpreting the results may be high, but without a good technical team able to deliver the highest quality results day after day, these are both worthless. The patients, and the referring clinicians, are entitled to expect the best technical quality from the test; this is, unfortunately, not always available. By writing this book, incorporating all his experience, Raman Mistry will be going some way to ensure that a larger number of patients get consistently good information from their diagnostic tests.

Nothing stands still in medicine, and there is no reason to believe that nuclear medicine will be an exception. In our department, we will go on developing this manual as methods are improved and new techniques are introduced. This manual incorporates what we have learned over the years, and it should provide a basis from which other departments can develop their service, particularly when they do not have access to a person who has devoted many years to nuclear medicine technology and to ensuring quality.

I personally have many reasons to be thankful to Raman Mistry, and not least of these is his ability to provide this quality on which our clinical work and reputation depend.

Professor M. N. Maisey
1988

ABBREVIATIONS

ACD	acid citrate dextrose
ASIS	anterior superior iliac spine
BP	blood pressure
BP	British Pharmacopoeia
CABG	coronary artery bypass graft
CAD	coronary artery disease
CCK	cholecystokinin
CSF	cerebrospinal fluid
DC	direct current
DMSA	dimercaptosuccinic acid
DTPA	diethylenetriaminepentaacetic acid
ECG	electrocardiograph
ED	end diastole
EDTA	ethylenediaminetetraacetic acid
ES	end systole
g	acceleration due to gravity
GAP	general all-purpose (collimator)
GFR	glomerular filtration rate
GHA	glucoheptonate
GI	gastrointestinal
HIDA	phenylcarbamoylmethyldiaminoacetic acid
HSA	human serum albumin
i.u.	international unit
IV	intravenously
LAO	left anterior oblique
LPO	left posterior oblique
LVEF	left ventricular ejection fraction
MAA	macroaggregated albumin
MDP	methylene diphosphonate
MIBG	*meta*-iodobenzylguanidine
PCV	packed cell volume
PPP	platelet-poor plasma

PYP	pyrophosphate
q.s.	*quantum sufficit* (a sufficient quantity)
RAO	right anterior oblique
RBC	red blood cell
RCV	red-cell volume
ROI	region of interest
rpm	revolutions per minute
RPO	right posterior oblique
R–R	interval between one maximum of the QRS complex and the next
SIJ	sacroiliac joint
SSN	suprasternal notch
SVC	superior vena cava
TG	thyroglobulin
TRH	thyrotropin-releasing hormone
TSH	thyroid-stimulating hormone (thyrotropin)
USP	United States Pharmacopoeia
VA	ventriculoatrial
VP	ventriculoperitoneal
VSD	ventriculoseptal defect
WBC	white blood cell

RADIONUCLIDES USABLE WITH GAMMA CAMERAS

Element	Nuclide	Physical half life	Principal gamma photopeak energy (keV)
Cobalt	^{57}Co	270 days	122
Gallium	^{67}Ga	78 hours	92/184/296
Indium	^{111}In	2.8 days	173/247
Iodine	^{131}I	8 days	364
Iodine	^{123}I	13 hours	159
Krypton	$^{81}Kr^{m}$	13 secs	190
Selenium	^{75}Se	120 days	136/265
Technetium	$^{99}Tc^{m}$	6 hours	140
Thallium	^{201}Tl	73 hours	70
Xenon	^{133}Xe	5.2 days	81

CHAPTER ONE

RENAL IMAGING STUDIES

INTRODUCTION

Two types of renal imaging studies are performed in nuclear medicine – static and dynamic.

$^{99}Tc^m$ Dimercaptosuccinic acid (DMSA) binds to renal tubules within 3 h following injection and is routinely used for static imaging. The images provide accurate information about number, size and position of the kidneys and is useful in patients with suspected tumours, cysts, and trauma. The oblique views are especially useful in detecting renal cortical scarring which is found in the paediatric population.

$^{99}Tc^m$ Diethylenetriaminepentaacetic acid (DTPA) is routinely used for dynamic renal imaging. It is cleared by the kidneys primarily through glomerular filtration and therefore measures GFR. The study provides information about relative renal blood flow, and obstruction. It may also be used to detect ureteric reflux and in the estimation of residual volume. A major current application is for the serial evaluation of patients after a renal transplant, to establish the integrity of the vascular supply cortical function and the integrity of the collecting systems.

$^{99}Tc^m$-DTPA is of particular value in patients with known or suspected allergy to iodine-containing contrast material when contrast radiography may not be possible.

The two-kidney renal study with frusemide washout is used to differentiate obstructive and non-obstructive hydronephrosis. In an obstructive hydronephrosis, washout of activity does not occur following the injection of frusemide while washout of activity occurs if no obstruction is present. Combined with low radiation dose, the frusemide washout test provides a safe and simple noninvasive procedure. These characteristics are important for repeated studies that may be necessary in children.

Vesicoureteric reflux is an important cause of recurrent urinary tract infections and non-obstructive hydronephrosis. The radionuclide renal reflux study may be used to both detect and follow-up patients with ureteric reflux.

There are a number of substances, the sole route of excretion of which is through the kidneys. One such agent is orthoiodohippurate. Labelled with ^{123}I, it provides a renal imaging agent which is cleared by both glomerular filtration and tubular secretion. Unfortunately, the cost of producing this agent makes its routine use uneconomical. It is therefore generally used selectively on patients with renal artery stenosis, for which it is best suited.

As well as qualitative data, quantitative information can be obtained from renal imaging studies, including differential function and transit times.

1.1 RADIOPHARMACEUTICALS

1.1.1 ^{99}Tc^m-DTPA(Sn)

> **Note**
> *Aseptic procedure*   Switch on the laminar flow cabinet at least 30 min before starting.

1. Collect the following:
    (a) one vial of DTPA kit
    (b) one lead pot
    (c) one 10 ml syringe with 21G (green) needle
    (d) ^{99}Tc^m-Pertechnetate of correct concentration
    (e) one swab (isopropyl alcohol or chlorhexidine)
2. Remove the central metal disc from the DTPA labelling vial.
3. Swab the rubber closures of the labelling and pertechnetate vials.
4. Place the labelling vial in the lead pot.
5. Transfer the activity and volume of pertechnetate, as recommended by the manufacturer, into the labelling vial. Withdraw an equal volume of gas from the vial.
6. Shake for 1 min.
7. Assay and label the vial with activity, volume, time, date, batch number and expiry time.
8. Record the following in the radiopharmaceutical records book:
    (a) date
    (b) name of preparation
    (c) manufacturer's lot number

(d) $^{99}Tc^m$ generator number
(e) total activity in vial
(f) volume
(g) time
(h) batch number

1.1.2 $^{99}Tc^m$-DMSA

> **Note.**
> *Aseptic procedure* Switch on the laminar flow cabinet at least 30 min before starting.

1. Collect the following:
   (a) one vial of DMSA kit
   (b) one lead pot
   (c) one 10 ml syringe with 21G (green) needle
   (d) $^{99}Tc^m$-pertechnetate of recommended concentration
   (e) one swab (isopropyl alcohol or chlorhexidine)
2. Remove the central metal disc from the DMSA labelling vial.
3. Swab the rubber closures of the labelling and pertechnetate vials.
4. Place the DMSA vial in the lead pot.
5. Transfer the activity and volume of pertechnetate, as recommended by the manufacturer, into the labelling vial.
6. Carefully withdraw an equal volume of gas from the vial. It is important not to allow oxygen into the vial.
7. Assay and label the vial with activity, volume, time, date, batch number and expiry time.
8. Use within the shelf-life and store as recommended by the manufacturer.
9. Record the following in the radiopharmaceutical records book:
   (a) date
   (b) name of preparation
   (c) manufacturer's lot number
   (d) $^{99}Tc^m$ generator number
   (e) total activity in vial
   (f) volume
   (g) time
   (h) batch number

1.1.3 ^{123}I-HIPPURAN

This is obtained ready for use, and the only procedure necessary is to check the activity against the label on the pot and the expiry time and date.

1.2 STANDARD DYNAMIC TWO-KIDNEY RENAL STUDY USING $^{99}Tc^m$-DTPA

1.2.1 PATIENT PREPARATION

The patient should be given 150–200 ml (two plastic beakers) of water to drink 15–30 min before the study in order to assure a relatively constant degree of hydration. If the patient is on fluid restriction, as may occur in patients in renal failure, this is not essential. If the patient's fluid intake is being recorded, ensure that the volume ingested is entered on the patient's fluid balance chart.

1.2.2 RADIOPHARMACEUTICAL AND DOSE

175 MBq $^{99}Tc^m$-DTPA

This is the adult dose, and should be corrected on the basis of body surface area in children and very large adults. For adults in renal failure, the dose is doubled. The minimum does is 75 MBq. In all cases the dose is injected as a bolus.

1.2.3 EQUIPMENT

A wide-field-of-view gamma camera, fitted with a general-purpose or high-resolution collimator, is used, connected to a computer. For children, the magnified mode ('Mag') is used on the camera and the computer if necessary.

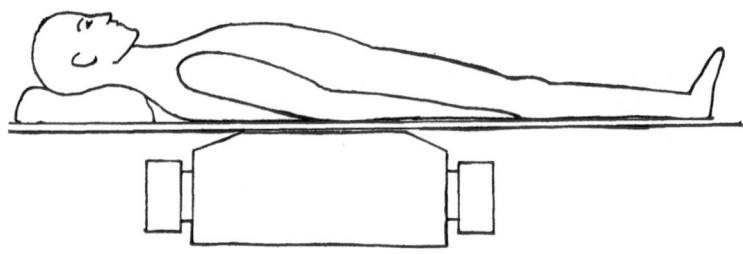

Fig. 1.1   Patient positioning for a two-kidney DTPA study.

1.2.4 PATIENT POSITIONING

The patient is positioned supine (Fig. 1.1) with pillows under the knees if the patient prefers this. In the case of babies, the child is placed directly on the camera face with an incontinence pad to avoid accidental contamination of the collimator. Two ^{57}Co marker sources (3.7 MBq each) are attached to the patient's sides in line with the lower costal margins, to assist positioning and to check for patient movement during analysis.

Remember to remove the marker sources at the end of the study.

1.2.5 COMPUTER

The computer is set up to record at one frame per 20 s in matrix 4 (64 × 64 word) for 20 min, i.e. a total of 60 frames.

1.2.6 TECHNIQUE

Injection technique

Attach a blood pressure cuff with Velcro fasteners above the patients' elbow in the arm to be used for injecting. Inflate the cuff to 100 mm of mercury and insert the needle in a suitable vein. Check that the needle is in position by drawing back a small amount of blood into the syringe. Increase the pressure to 200 mm of mercury, inject the contents of the syringe slowly into the vein and rapidly release the cuff by pulling apart the Velcro bands. Ensure that the patient breathes normally, otherwise the bolus is likely to get fragmented.

Note

In patients with fistulae, it is advisable to use the saline flush technique of bolus administration (see Section 7.6.6). The fistula should not be used unless absolutely necessary.

---

1. Ensure patient has emptied bladder before positioning. Position the patient so that the arm to be used for injection is closest to the operator, i.e. away from the camera stand.
2. Set clock for 20 min.
3. Ensure computer, camera and film back or multiformatter are set.
4. Give bolus injection of ^{99}Tc^m-DTPA, starting camera and computer at moment of cuff release.
5. Record the first image on camera for 30 s (image 1).
6. At 1 min after injection, record image for 400 000 counts (image 2). Note the time taken for this image on the patient's request form for later

reference in case a delayed view needs to be recorded, so that a correction can be made for the physical decay of $^{99}Tc^m$.

7. At 5, 10 and 20 min, take images (3–5) for same length of time as taken for the 1 min image.
8. The patient is then asked to walk about for 5 min and then to empty the bladder. In the case of infants who are sedated, ask the parent or nurse accompanying the child to hold the patient upright for a few minutes. Following this, record the final image on position 6 to determine whether a frusemide study should be performed.
9. If a frusemide study is not indicated, the patient should then be advised to empty the bladder, and to keep drinking as much as possible for the next 2 h. This will help to reduce the radiation dose to the bladder.

1.2.7 IMAGE LAYOUT

1 0–30 s	**2** 1 min
3 5 min	**4** 10 min
5 20 min	**6** Post walk and micturation

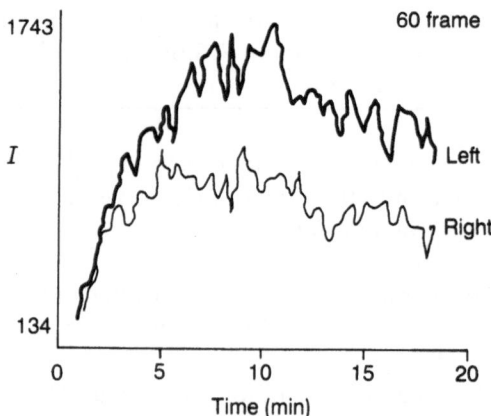

Fig. 1.2   Time–activity curves from a two-kidney DTPA study.

1.2.8 ANALYSIS

The aim of the analysis is to generate functional ('renogram') curves using regions of interests drawn around each of the kidneys, and to estimate the divided function from the relative uptake at 2 min into the study.

The final display should show the two renal time–activity curves, with their respective background curves subtracted (Fig. 1.2) together with an image displaying the regions of interest (ROI) drawn on it.

Two sets of hard-copy prints should be recorded, one for sending out with the patient's report and one for retaining in the scan envelope.

1.3 TWO-KIDNEY RENAL STUDY USING FRUSEMIDE DIURESIS

1.3.1 PATIENT PREPARATION

The patient will have had a standard two-kidney renal study performed. Ask the patient to walk about for a few minutes and then to go and empty the bladder. In the case of infants who are sedated, ask the parent or nurse to hold the patient upright for a few minutes. Position patient so that both the kidneys and bladder are in the field of view. Record an image for the same length of time as in renal study and show it to the doctor on duty to see if a frusemide study is indicated.

1.3.2 RADIOPHARMACEUTICAL

In children, the dose of frusemide used depends on the weight of the child:

For children weighing less than 10 kg, use 2 mg/kg
For children weighing more than 10 kg, use 20 mg
The standard *adult* dose is 0.5 mg/kg

In all cases the frusemide is injected intravenously.

1.3.3 EQUIPMENT

Ideally the same camera as was used for the two-kidney renal study should be used, but any other camera fitted with a general-purpose or high-resolution collimator may be used.

1.3.4 PATIENT POSITIONING

The patient is positioned as in the two-kidney renal study, but with both the kidneys and the bladder in the field of view.
   Remember to remove the marker sources at the end of the study.

1.3.5 COMPUTER

The computer is set up to record one frame every 20 s in matrix 4 (64 × 64 word) for 10 min, i.e. a total of 30 frames.

1.3.6 TECHNIQUE

1. Ensure the computer is set.

2. Set clock for 10 min.
3. Ensure camera, film back and multiformatter are set.
4. Start camera and computer acquisition just before or as frusemide is injected.
5. Record successive images at 2, 5 and 10 min for the same length of time as in the two-kidney renal study.
6. At the end of the study, record an image to include the bladder if the bladder is not visible on the other images.
7. The patient should then be advised to empty the bladder, and to keep drinking as much as possible for the next 2 h. This will help to reduce the radiation dose to the bladder.

1.3.7 IMAGE LAYOUT

0 min	2 min
5 min	10 min
	(Bladder)

1.3.8 ANALYSIS

The aim of the analysis is to generate functional curves from each kidney, and to calculate the half-time of washout from each kidney following the injection of frusemide. Using irregular regions of interest (ROI), the right and left pelves are outlined and time–activity curves are generated (Fig. 1.3).

Calculation of washout fraction

Washout fractions are calculated as follows:

$$\text{Washout from right kidney (\%)} = \frac{R(max) - R(min)}{R(max)} \times 100$$

$$\text{Washout from left kidney (\%)} = \frac{L(max) - L(min)}{L(max)} \times 100$$

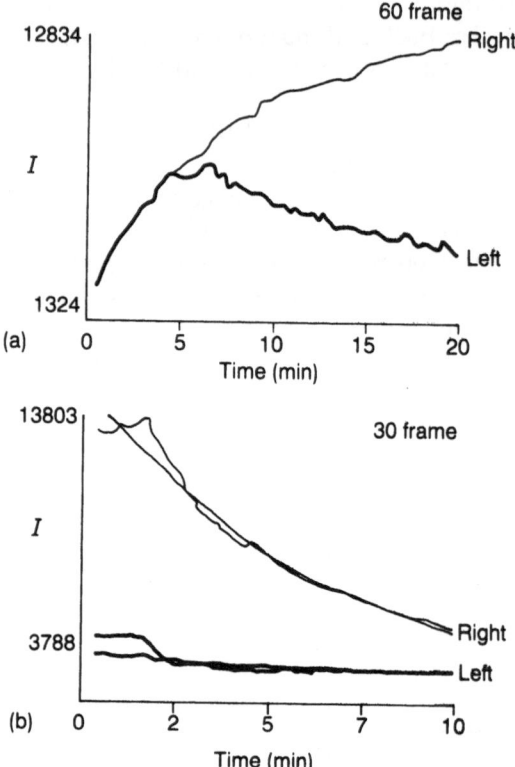

Fig. 1.3   Time–activity curves from a two-kidney renal frusemide washout study: (a) right GFR 48.8%, left GFR 51.2%; (b) right washout 71.3%, left washout 50.6%, right half-time 4.8 min, left half-time 13.4 min.

where R(max) = counts from maximum on right pelvic ROI curve, R(min) = counts from minimum point on right pelvic ROI curve, L(max) = counts from maximum point on left pelvic ROI curve and L(min) = counts from minimum point on left pelvic ROI curve.

The half-time, in minutes, of clearance is calculated by fitting an exponential function to each curve.

1.4 URETERIC REFLUX STUDY

1.4.1 PATIENT PREPARATION

The patient will have had a standard DTPA two-kidney renal study. Following this, the patient should have been asked to drink as much as possible and report back to the technician when the patient has a desire to micturate.

1.4.2 RADIOPHARMACEUTICAL

$^{99}Tc^m$-DTPA

This is injected at the start of the two-kidney renal study.

1.4.3 EQUIPMENT

The study is performed on the standard-field-of-view camera, fitted with the gap collimator or diverging collimator if necessary. A wide-field-of-view camera may also be used but should be placed on 'Mag' for imaging children. A suitably adapted commode is a worthwhile investment, as many of the patients are children.

1.4.4 PATIENT POSITIONG

To maintain privacy, the patient should be screened off using mobile screens. Attach two ^{57}Co markers posteriolaterally on the costal margins.

Girls should· be positioned sitting on a bedpan on a chair or the commode, with their back as close as possible to the camera face.

Boys should be positioned to stand with their back touching the camera and given a bedpan or urinal, or a commode can be used.

Both the kidneys and bladder should be well within the field of view of the camera. The camera height should be adjusted so that the bladder appears at the bottom of the field of view.

1.4.5 COMPUTER

The computer is set up to record at one frame per 10 s for 300 s using a 64 × 64 word matrix. The total number of frames will be 30.

1.4.6 TECHNIQUE

1. When the patient expresses a desire to micturate, position the patient in front of the camera as in patient positioning and start recording. Note the time at which it is started. A 2 min baseline should be recorded before asking the patient to micturate.
2. At the end of the 2 min, instruct the patient to micturate when ready, and

monitor the performance on the persistence scope. Note the time taken to empty the bladder.

> **Note**
> No images are recorded during the study, in order to minimize disturbing the patient.

3. When the patient has finished micturating, the data acquisition should be allowed to run for a further 2 min.
4. The patient should then be advised to keep drinking as much as possible for the next 2 h. This will help to reduce the radiation dose to the bladder.

1.4.7 ANALYSIS

The aim of the analysis is to generate and display curves generated from pelves regions of interest to indicate whether there is any increase in counts with micturition, indicating reflux (Fig. 1.4).

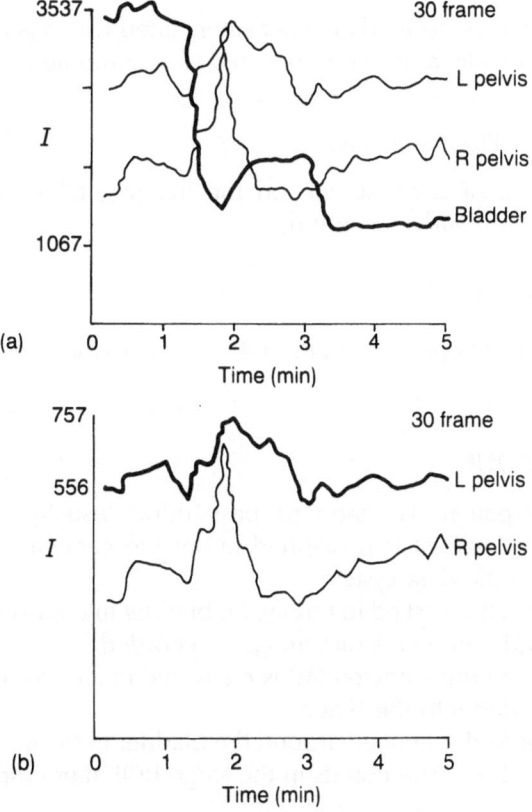

Fig. 1.4 Time–activity curves from a ureteric reflux study.

1.5 RESIDUAL BLADDER VOLUME ESTIMATION

1.5.1 PATIENT PREPARATION

No specific preparation is needed, but it may be helpful to give 200 ml (two plastic beakers) of water to drink. The study may be performed after a standard two-kidney, transplant or reflux study without any preparation.

1.5.2 RADIOPHARMACEUTICAL AND DOSE

35 MBq $^{99}Tc^m$-DTPA(Sn)

This is a standard dose for all patients (unless it is part of a standard DTPA renal study).

1.5.3 EQUIPMENT

The study may be performed on any camera fitted with a general-purpose or high-resolution collimator and connected to a computer.

1.5.4 PATIENT POSITIONING

The patient is positioned supine on the imaging table with the camera centred over the bladder, anteriorly.

1.5.5 COMPUTER

The computer is set up to record in a 64 × 64 word matrix for 1 min for each of the two images.

1.5.6 TECHNIQUE

1. When the patient is ready to pass urine (usually about 1 h after injection),the patient is positioned under the camera and the image is recorded on the data system.
2. The patient is then asked to empty the bladder into a disposable urinal or bedpan, and a further 1 min image is recorded.
3. The volume of urine passed (M) is measured in a measuring jug, and the urine discarded into the sluice.
4. An irregular ROI is defined around the bladder in the first image, and the counts noted (A). The counts in the same ROI after emptying are noted (B).

Calculation of residual volume

The residual bladder volume is calculated as:

$$\text{Residual volume (ml)} = M \times \frac{B}{A-B}$$

where M = volume of urine passed, A = counts in bladder before micturition and B = counts in same bladder region after micturition.

1.6 TWO-KIDNEY RENAL STUDY USING ^{123}I-HIPPURAN

This study is usually performed in screening patients with hypertension or unilateral renal disease.

1.6.1 PATIENT PREPARATION

The patient is given 150–200 ml (two plastic beakers) of water to drink 15–30 min before the study in order to assure a relatively constant degree of hydration. If the patient is on fluid restriction, as may occur in patients in renal failure, this is not essential. If the patient's fluid intake is being recorded ensure that the volume drunk is entered on the patient's fluid balance chart. The patient should be asked to empty the bladder immediately before the study starts.

1.6.2 RADIOPHARMACEUTICAL AND DOSE

35 MBq ^{123}I-hippuran

This is a standard dose for all patients.

1.6.3 EQUIPMENT

A large-field-of-view camera is used with a general-purpose or a high-resolution collimator. If the ^{123}I is not pure, i.e. if it contains contaminants such as ^{124}I, then the medium-energy collimator should be used, otherwise the images will display a dark hexagon or circle along the edge of the field of view on some collimators.

1.6.4 PATIENT POSITIONING

The patient is positioned supine, with pillows to support the legs if the patient prefers it. To ensure correct positioning, ^{57}Co markers are attached bilaterally on the patient's costal margin so that they appear just above the midline of the persistence scope. If the patient is unable to lie supine, an imaging chair may be used.

1.6.5 COMPUTER

The computer is set up to record at one frame per 20 s using a 64 × 64 word matrix for 20 min. The total number of frames will be 60.

1.6.6 TECHNIQUE

1. Ensure the computer is set.
2. Set clock for 20 min.
3. Ensure camera, film back and multiformatter are set.
4. Start acquisition on camera and computer as the intravenous injection is given.
5. Record the first image on the camera for 30 s (image 1).
6. At 1 min after injection, record image for 300 000 counts (image 2). Note the time taken for this image.
7. At 5, 10 and 20 min, take images (3–5) for same time as taken to record the 1 min image.
8. At 20 min, take posterior image of bladder or catheter bag (6). This must be done, even if no counts are present, for later reference.
9. The patient should then be advised to empty the bladder, and to keep drinking as much as possible for the next 2 h. This will help to reduce the radiation dose to the bladder.

1.6.7 IMAGE LAYOUT

1 0–30 s	2 1 min
3 5 min	4 10 min
5 20 min	6 Bladder

1.6.8 ANALYSIS

The purpose of the analysis is to generate functional ('renogram') curves for each kidney, and then to display them to see whether there is any delay in time of peak, such as is found in renal artery stenosis (Fig. 1.5). Parenchymal transit times are also calculated in patients with abnormal studies.

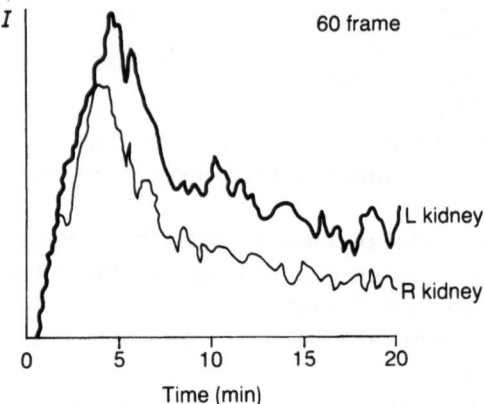

Fig. 1.5   Time–activity curves from a two-kidney ^{123}I-hippuran study.

1.7 RENAL TRANSPLANT STUDY

1.7.1 PATIENT PREPARATION

The patient is asked to drink 150–200 ml (two plastic beakers) of water 15–30 min before the study in order to assure a relatively constant degree of hydration. If the patient is on fluid restriction, as may occur in the early phase after transplantation, this is not essential. If the patient's fluid intake is being recorded, ensure that the drink is entered on the fluid balance chart. The patient should be asked to empty the bladder immediately before starting the study.

1.7.2 RADIOPHARMACEUTICAL AND DOSE

350 MBq $^{99}Tc^m$-DTPA

This is the adult dose, and should be corrected on the basis of body surface area in children and very large adults. The minimum dose is 75 MBq.

The study may also be performed using $^{99}Tc^m$-MDP if the patient is having a bone study.

1.7.3 EQUIPMENT

A wide-field-of-view gamma camera, fitted with a general-purpose or high-resolution collimator, is used, connected to a computer.

1.7.4 PATIENT POSITIONING

The patient is positioned supine (Fig. 1.6) with the camera positioned anteriorly over the abdomen. A large-field camera is used; therefore, in

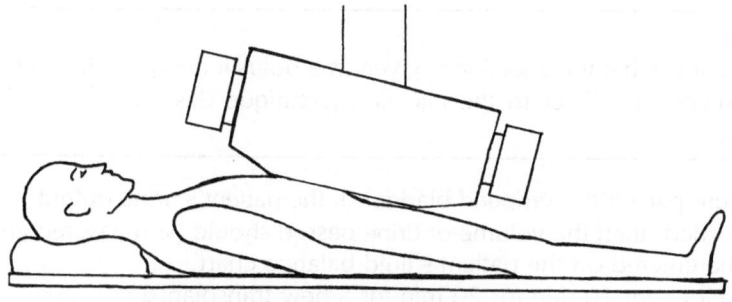

Fig. 1.6   Patient positioning for a renal transplant study.

children, it must be set to 'Mag'. To maintain consistency, the same camera should be used for all follow up studies on the same patient.

For reproducibility, a ^{57}Co marker should be placed on the patient's umbilicus and the patient should be positioned so that the marker is opposite the upper edge of the side of the hexagon and halfway between the apex and side on the side away from the transplant, as seen on the persistence scope:

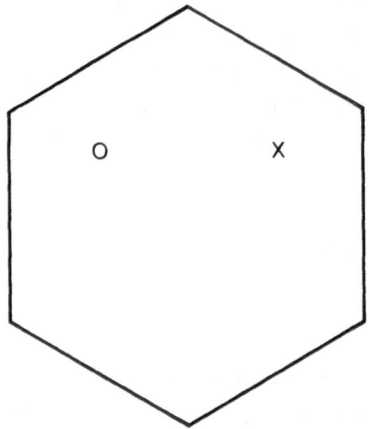

Here O indicates the position of the marker on the persistence scope for left-sided transplant and X indicates the position for right-sided transplant.

1.7.5 COMPUTER

The computer is set up to record at one frame per second on a 64 × 64 byte matrix for 30 s, and then one frame per minute in a 64 × 64 word matrix for 10 min, i.e. a total of 40 frames.

1.7.6 TECHNIQUE

> **Note**
> It is critical that the injection is given as a bolus if the quantitation is to be successful. Refer to the injection technique described in Section 1.2.6.

1. Ensure patient has emptied bladder. If the patient's urine output is being recorded, then the volume of urine passed should be measured and the value entered on the patient's fluid balance chart.
2. Set clock for 10 min (or 20 min for a new transplant).
3. Ensure computer, camera and film back are set.

4. Give bolus injection of $^{99}Tc^m$-DTPA, starting camera and computer at moment of cuff release.
5. Record first image on camera for 30 s (1).
6. At 1 min after injection, record image for 400 000 counts (2). Note the time taken for this image on the patient's request form for later reference in case a delayed view is necessary.
7. At 5, 10 (15) and 20 min, take images (image positions 3–5) for same time as taken for 1 min image.
8. At 20 min, record an anterior image of the bladder or catheter bag (image position 6). This must be done, even if no counts are present, for later reference.
9. The patient should then be advised to empty the bladder, and to keep drinking as much as is allowed for the next 2 h. This will help to reduce the radiation dose to the bladder.

1.7.7 IMAGE LAYOUT

1 0–30 s	2 1 min
3 5 min	4 10 min
5 20 min	6 Bladder

1.7.8 ANALYSIS

The purpose of the analysis is to generate time–activity curves using regions of interest drawn over the iliac artery distal to the transplant, around the transplanted kidney, and over a background region (Fig. 1.7). From these curves, a perfusion index is generated, as well as an index of renal uptake at 2 min. The curves also give information about transit and possible obstruction.

Several methods of quantifying the flow index have been suggested. One of them is that expressed as arterial counts per cell integrated to the peak and divided by concurrent renal counts per cell. Both the curves are background-subtracted. The value thus obtained is multiplied by 100 to give a whole number.

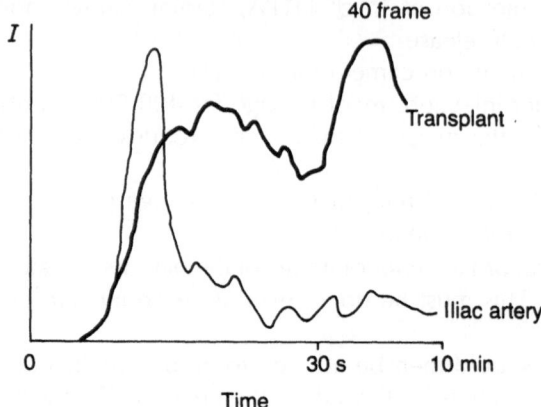

Fig. 1.7 Time–activity curves from a renal transplant study. Both curves are normalized, and the background is subtracted.

1.8 STATIC RENAL STUDY USING ^{99}Tc^m-DMSA

1.8.1 PATIENT PREPARATION

A small number of children may need to be sedated for the imaging section of the study, if the study is to be carried out efficiently. The need for sedation should be established at the time of injection.

1.8.2 RADIOPHARMACEUTICAL AND DOSE

200 MBq ^{99}Tc^m-DMSA

This is the adult dose and should be corrected on the basis of body surface area in children. The minimum dose is 37 MBq.

1.8.3 EQUIPMENT

A standard or wide-field-of-view gamma camera fitted with a high-resolution or general-purpose collimator is used, connected to a computer. The computer end should be fitted with a variable-gain control unit.

1.8.4 PATIENT POSITIONING

The patient is positioned supine with the camera positioned underneath the imaging table for the posterior and oblique views and above the patient for the anterior view. For oblique views, the 'giant wedge' or pillows are used to support the patient's back.

For babies, the child is placed directly over the camera face. An incontinence pad should be used to prevent possible contamination of the camera face.

Using patient monitor or persistence on the data system, adjust the gain to magnify the field of view and adjust the patient's position so that both the kidneys are just within the magnified field of view. Allow enough room to draw the background region of interest during analysis.

1.8.5 COMPUTER

The computer is set up to record each image for 300 s in a 64 × 64 word matrix, closing on overflow.

1.8.6 TECHNIQUE

1. The patient waits for a minimum of 3 h after intravenous injection of $^{99}Tc^m$-DMSA and should be warned about this when the study is booked. Patients in renal failure should be injected early in the morning and scanned as late as possible in the afternoon.
2. Position the patient as described under patient positioning.
3. Ensure the computer is set.
4. Record image on film for 650 000 counts. Do not move the patient until the computer acquisition stops.
5. Repeat steps 2, 3 and 4 for oblique and anterior views. For recording the anterior view, the camera must be positioned above the patient. The patient must not be positioned prone with the camera underneath the table for this anterior view, as the kidneys may become proptosed, making the analysis useless.

    The posterior view should be recorded with a ^{57}Co marker source positioned adjacent to the patient's right side. Do not leave the marker source there for too long since the computer acquisition is set to terminate on overflow.

1.8.7 IMAGE LAYOUT

Anterior	Posterior + ^{57}Co marker on right
Left posterior oblique	Right posterior oblique

1.8.8 ANALYSIS

The aim of the analysis is to calculate divided renal function, as a percentage of total renal function.

1. Select the anterior view.
2. Using irregular regions of interest, outline the right kidney, left kidney and a background region of interest (ideally a program should be written that automatically draws a background region of interest around each kidney, one pixel wide).
3. Repeat this procedure for the posterior view.

Calculation of geometric-mean estimation

Background-subtract each kidney in view. The background region should be normalized in terms of size to that of each corresponding renal region. Then calculate the following:

Counts left = $\sqrt{(AL \times PL)}$
Counts right = $\sqrt{(AR \times PR)}$

where AR = counts from right kidney in the anterior view, AL = counts from left kidney in the anterior view, PR = counts from right kidney in the posterior view and PL = counts from left kidney in the posterior view.

The geometric-mean divided function is then given by:

$$\text{Right kidney (\%)} = \frac{\text{Counts right}}{\text{Counts right} + \text{Counts left}} \times 100$$

$$\text{Left kidney (\%)} = \frac{\text{Counts left}}{\text{Counts right} + \text{Counts left}} \times 100$$

Calculation of arithmetic-mean estimation

The arithmetic-mean divided function is calculated by using the data from the posterior view only and background subtraction:

$$\text{Right kidney (\%)} = \frac{PR}{PR + PL} \times 100$$

$$\text{Left kidney (\%)} = \frac{PL}{PR + PL} \times 100$$

CHAPTER TWO

GLOMERULAR FILTRATION RATE

Introduction

Glomerular filtration rate (GFR) is a basic parameter of renal function. Its measurement is usually performed to determine renal clearance for evaluation and follow-up of renal disease. ^{51}Cr-Ethylenediaminetetraacetate (^{51}Cr-EDTA) is eliminated from the body only by glomerular filtration and thus clearance of this agent can be used to measure GFR. The method described provides a simple and accurate method to measure this parameter.

The patient should not have other nuclear medicine studies for several days prior to this measurement with the exception of ^{99}Tc^m-DTPA or ^{99}Tc^{m}DMSA renal imaging studies. If necessary, these can be performed simultaneously, but the GFR samples should be left for 48 h to allow for the decay of ^{99}Tc^m before sample counting.

2.1 DILUTION AND DISPENSING OF ^{51}Cr-EDTA

2.1.1 ADULT'S PREPARATION

This produces an activity of approximately 3 MBq/10 ml, which is suitable for patients aged 12 years and over.

> **Note**
> *Aseptic procedure*   Switch on the laminar flow cabinet at least 30 min before start of the procedure. Swab the cabinet with chlorhexidine 0.5% in 70% spirit before starting.

2.1.2 FORMULA

^{51}Cr-EDTA, 37 MBq/10 ml	111 MBq (nominal)
Benzyl alcohol 1% v/v and	
disodium edetate 0.1% w/v (pharmacy)	360 ml

2.1.3 MATERIALS

1. 111 MBq ^{51}Cr-EDTA solution.
2. 360 ml benzyl alcohol 1% v/v and disodium edetate 0.1% w/v (pharmacy)
3. One luer-luer connector.
4. Laboratory stand with clamp.
5. 20 ml syringes.
6. Five 21G (green) needles.
7. Two millipore filters (0.22 μm).
8. One butterfly needle (19G).
9. Thirty-five 15 ml sterile, pyrogen-free evacuated vials.

2.1.4 PROCEDURE FOR ADULT'S PREPARATION

1. Swab all items with chlorhexidine 0.5% in 70% alcohol before starting.
2. Transfer 111 MBq of ^{51}Cr-EDTA solution into the bottle of EDTA solution, using the 20 ml syringe, to give approximately 111 MBq ^{51}Cr-EDTA in 390 ml. Mix well.
3. Attach a millipore filter to the end of the butterfly. Insert the butterfly through the rubber stopper of the diluted ^{51}Cr-EDTA bottle. Allow 20 s for the pressure in the bottle to become atmospheric.

4. Invert the bottle, keeping the millipore filter above the level of the solution to avoid wetting it. Clamp in this position, keeping the millipore filter above the solution level.
5. Assemble the second millipore and luer-luer adaptor, and attach a green needle to each end. Insert one needle through stopper of the bottle, with the adaptor above the millipore.
6. Allow the solution to drain into the millipore under gravity, and, when the filter surface is completely covered with solution, attach the first evacuated vial.
7. Proceed until the solution is completely dispensed, ensuring that each vial contains at least 12 ml.
8. Label each vial with the activity, volume, time and date of preparation, batch number and expiry date (two weeks from the preparation date).
9. Rinse the empty bottle three times with water and pour washings carefully into the designated waste disposal sluice, then flush away. All active syringes, needles and millipore filters must be stored in a lead pot in a designated cupboard until the activity has decayed.
10. Record the following in the ^{51}Cr-EDTA record book on a fresh sheet:
    (a) date and time of preparation
    (b) batch number of preparation (series COAD 2000 for adults)
    (c) initials of technician
    (d) expiry date
    (e) ingredients (including batch number and expiry date of millipore filters, butterfly, ^{51}Cr-EDTA and EDTA solution (pharmacy)

2.1.5 CHILD'S AND INFANT'S PREPARATION

This produces an activity of approximately 2 MBq/10 ml, which is suitable for patients aged 3–12 years, and of approximately 1 MBq/5 ml, which is suitable for infants up to 3 years in age.

Note
Aseptic procedure   Switch on the laminar flow cabinet at least 30 min before start of procedure. Swab cabinet with chlorhexidine 0.5% in 70% spirit before starting

---

2.1.6 FORMULA

^{51}Cr-EDTA, 37MBq/10 ml	75 MBq (nominal)
Benzyl alcohol 1% v/v and	
disodium edetate 0.1% w/v (pharmacy)	360 ml

2.1.7 MATERIALS

1. 75 MBq ^{51}Cr-EDTA solution.
2. 360 ml benzyl alcohol 1% v/v and disodium edetate 0.1% w/v (pharmacy).
3. One luer-luer connector.
4. Laboratory stand with clamp.
5. 20 ml syringes.
6. Five 21G (green) needles.
7. Two millipore filters (0.22 μm).
8. One butterfly needle (19G).
9. Thirty-five 15 ml sterile, pyrogen-free evacuated vials.

2.1.8 PROCEDURE FOR CHILD'S AND INFANT'S PREPARATION

1. Swab all items with chlorhexidine 0.5% in 70% alcohol before starting.
2. Transfer 75 MBq of ^{51}Cr-EDTA solution into the bottle of EDTA solution using the 20 ml syringe to give approximately 75 MBq ^{51}Cr-EDTA in 370 ml. Mix well.
3. Attach a millipore filter to the end of the butterfly. Insert the butterfly through the rubber stopper of the diluted ^{51}Cr-EDTA bottle. Allow 20 s for the pressure in the bottle to become atmospheric.
4. Invert the bottle, keeping the millipore filter above the level of the solution to avoid wetting it. Clamp in this position, keeping the millipore filter above the solution level.
5. Assemble the second millipore and luer-luer adaptor, and attach a green needle to each end. Insert one needle through the stopper of the bottle, with the adaptor above the millipore.
6. Allow the solution to drain into the millipore under gravity, and, when the filter surface is completely covered with solution, attach the first evacuated vial.
7. Proceed until the solution is completely dispensed, ensuring that each vial contains at least 12 ml for the child's preparation and 6 ml for the infant's.
8. Label each vial with the activity, volume, time and date of preparation, batch number and expiry date (four weeks from the preparation date).
9. Rinse the empty bottle three times with water and pour washings carefully into the designated waste disposal sluice, then flush away. All active syringes, needles and millipore filters must be stored in a lead pot in a designated cupboard until the activity has decayed.
10. Record the following in the ^{51}Cr-EDTA record book on a fresh sheet: (a) date and time of preparation.

(b) batch number of preparation (series COCH 1000 for child's doses and COIN 1000 for infant's doses)
(c) initials of technician
(d) expiry date
(e) ingredients (including batch number and expiry date of millipore filters, butterfly, ^{51}Cr-EDTA and EDTA solution (pharmacy))

2.2 TECHNIQUE OF GFR ESTIMATION USING ^{51}Cr-EDTA

2.2.1 TECHNIQUE

No patient preparation is required, but the patient ideally should not have other nuclear medicine studies for several days prior to this measurement.

Inject exactly 5 or 10 ml (depending on age) of the dilute ^{51}Cr-EDTA solution intravenously. This should be done accurately using a 5 or 10 ml syringe, filling it exactly to the mark and then injecting the contents completely. Flush the syringe. Note the exact time of injection.

The remainder of the dilute ^{51}Cr-EDTA solution is kept for preparation of the standard.

At 2, 3 and 4 h after injection, take 5–10 ml samples from the opposite arm into 10 ml heparinized tubes. Do not use 2 or 5 ml tubes. The exact volume of the sample does not matter. Note the time of the samples, using the same watch or clock used for recording the time of injection.

If the patient's renal function is moderately impaired, take samples at 2, 3, 4 and 6 h. If the renal function is likely to be severely impaired or the patient is oedematous, samples should be taken at 3, 6, 9 and 12 h. Table 2.1 shows a typical form used for GFR estimation.

Note
The critical points are to inject exactly 5 or 10 ml, and to note all times accurately using the same watch or clock.

2.2.2 SAMPLE PREPARATION AND SAMPLING

1. Spin the samples for 5 min at 2500 rpm (5.5 g).
2. From each sample, accurately pipette 3.0 ml plasma into a 10 ml tube marked with the patients' name and the sample number. The same pipette may be used for all three samples, provided that the samples are pipetted in reverse order. If the samples are not large enough, use the maximum plasma volume provided and correct the counts for different volumes. Before counting, the low-volume samples should be made

equal in volume to the large samples by adding distilled water, in order to maintain consistent counting geometry.

Table 2.1   Typical form used for GFR estimation.

Department of Nuclear Medicine Measurement of glomerula filtration rate using ^{51}Cr-EDTA		
Height	cm	Ward
Weight	kg	Surname
		First name
Batch no.		Unit no.
		Date of birth

Clinical details

Date   Signature

Instructions
1. All the details on this form *must* be completed in full!
2. There are three dilutions of ^{51}Cr-EDTA – for adults, children (3–12 years) and infants (under 3 years). These have different serial numbers and labels. Be sure to use the correct preparation
3. Inject the correct volume of ^{51}Cr-EDTA intravenously (10 ml for adults and children, 5 ml for infants) using a 10 ml or a 5 ml syringe and record the exact time on the form.
4. Take 10 ml heparinized blood samples at approximately 2, 3 and 4 h after injection from the opposite arm to that into which the injection was given. If renal function is moderately impaired or the patient is oedematous, sample at 2, 3, 4 and 6 h; if it is severely impaired, sample at 3, 4, 6 and 12 h.
5. Record the exact times of injection and sampling on the form and on the samples. The intervals are not critical but the times are.
6. Return the blood samples, this form and the ^{51}Cr-EDTA bottle to the Nuclear Medicine Dept as soon as possible.
7. ^{51}Cr-EDTA is radioactive; any surplus should be returned to the bottle. Use it immediately – don't store it 'in case'.
8. If you have any queries, please ring the Nuclear Medicine Dept.

Time of injection		*Laboratory use only*	Vol.
Time of first sample		Bgrd	Std
Time of second sample			
Time of third sample			
Time of fourth sample			
Time of fifth sample			

2.2.3 PREPARATION OF THE STANDARD

Dispense 1 ml of the remaining ^{51}Cr-EDTA for the adult's and child's batches and 0.5 ml for the infant's batches into separate 250 ml volumetric flasks. Make the volume up to 250 ml with distilled water. Pipette an equal volume of the standard solution into a 10 ml tube, to be counted with the samples.

Note
Infant's standard may be counted using the child's standard and using 5 ml injection volume for calculation.

2.2.4 COUNTING

Count each sample, the standard and a background tube for 1000 s, on a ^{51}Cr window.

2.2.5 CALCULATION

1. Correct the counts of each sample for background and volumes if samples were of different volumes.
2. Plot corrected counts against time on semi-log paper.
3. Calculate $T_{1/2}$ in min and intercept at time 0 (initial count rate).
4. Then calculate

$$VD \, (l) = \frac{S \times D \times V}{A \times 1000}$$

   where VD = volume of distribution in litres, S = count rate of standard (background-corrected), D = dilution of standard, V = volume injected in ml and A = count rate at time 0 (obtained from intercept at time 0).
5. Then the GFR is given by:

$$GFR \, (ml/min) = \frac{VD \times 1000 \times 0.693 \times 0.87}{T_{1/2}}$$

   where GFR is the glomerular filtration rate in millilitres per minute.
6. The result is corrected to a surface area of 1.73 m^2 via

$$\text{Corrected GFR} = GFR \times \frac{1.73}{\text{Patient's body surface area}}$$

CHAPTER THREE

BONE IMAGING STUDIES

Introduction

Bone imaging is now one of the most reliable, sensitive and cost effective procedures in nuclear medicine and forms a major portion of any nuclear medicine workload. There are many bone imaging agents available which can be labelled with $^{99}Tc^m$, most commonly used of which is $^{99}Tc^m$ methylene diphosphonate (MDP).

Areas of bone injury or bone destruction are usually associated with bone repair, with increased metabolic activity and increased bone flow. This increased metabolic bone activity results in $^{99}Tc^m$-labelled bone-seeking radiopharmaceuticals being deposited in these regions of bone repair in higher concentrations relative to normal bone.

Bone imaging is generally more sensitive than conventional X-rays in detecting the presence and extent of active bone pathology and is most frequently used in detecting bone metastases. Follow-up imaging is routinely performed to monitor the effects of therapy.

In stress fractures, osteomyelitis and Legg–Perthe's disease, the bone scan is positive before conventional X-rays as scan changes frequently precede X-ray changes. Bone imaging is also useful in metabolic disorders such as Paget's disease and hyperparathyroidism.

Dynamic imaging combined with static imaging at 4 h is extremely useful in diagnosing stress fractures, evaluating hip and knee prostheses and also for determination of vascularity of the femoral head as an aid in establishing the diagnosis of ankylosing spondylitis.

Bone imaging is also used in the confirmation and evaluation of non-accidental injury (NAI) or the battered child syndrome.

As with all other nuclear medicine imaging procedures, contamination of the patient's skin or clothing can cause image artefacts and this should always be borne in mind, particularly when imaging the young and the elderly.

Rotating gamma camera tomography has also been found to be useful in evaluating conditions such as avascular necrosis. Other non-routine views such as the 'outlet' view and oblique views of the spine provide additional information in some cases.

3.1 RADIOPHARMACEUTICALS

3.1.1 $^{99}Tc^m$-MDP

> **Note**
> *Aseptic procedure*   Switch on the laminar flow cabinet at least 30 min before starting. Swab with 0.5% chlorhexidine in 70% spirit.

1. Collect the following:
   - (a) one vial of MDP kit
   - (b) one lead pot
   - (c) one 10 ml syringe with 21G (green) needle
   - (d) $^{99}Tc^m$-pertechnetate having the desired activity
   - (e) one swab (isopropyl alcohol or chlorhexidine)
2. Remove the central metal disc from the MDP labelling vial.
3. Swab the rubber closures of the labelling and pertechnetate vials.
4. Place the labelling vial in the lead pot.
5. Transfer $^{99}Tc^m$-pertechnetate, maximum activity 18 000 MBq (in 2–8 ml), into the labelling vial. Withdraw an equal volume of gas from the vial.
6. Shake gently for 1 min.
7. Measure the activity and label the vial with activity, volume, time, date, batch number and expiry time.
8. Use within 6 h of preparation.
9. Record the following in the radiopharmaceutical records book:
   - (a) date
   - (b) name of preparation
   - (c) manufacturer's lot number
   - (d) $^{99}Tc^m$ generator number
   - (e) total activity in vial
   - (f) volume
   - (g) time
   - (h) batch number

3.2 ROUTINE BONE IMAGING

3.2.1 PATIENT PREPARATION

The patient is advised to increase fluid intake for the rest of the day following the injection. This will help to reduce the radiation dosage to the bladder and also help improve the image quality by reducing the soft-tissue count rate.

Some children may need to be sedated for the imaging part of the study, and this should be decided at the time of injection.

3.2.2 RADIOPHARMACEUTICAL AND DOSE

550 MBq ^{99}Tc^m-MDP

This is the adult dose and is adjusted in relation to body surface area in children and very large adults.

3.2.3 PATIENT POSITIONING

All images are recorded with the patient lying on the imaging table. Anterior images are recorded with the patient supine, and posterior images are recorded with the patient prone (Fig. 3.1). The camera is only placed under the imaging table if the patient is unable to lie prone.

3.2.4 EQUIPMENT

The study is performed on a large-field-of-view camera using a general-purpose or high-resolution collimator.

3.2.5 COMPUTER

A computer is necessary for sacroiliac quantitation studies and for recording bone flow studies. If the facilities are available, it may be used for backing up all the routine images. The digital images can then be recorded on photographic paper for sending out with the patient's scan reports.

3.2.6 TECHNIQUE

1. Ensure patient has emptied bladder.
2. Ensure camera and film back or multiformatter are set.

3. Begin by recording the dorsal spine view for 500 000 counts (750 000 or 5 min if using wider-field cameras).
4. Record further views following the image layout below using the preset time noted on the first image.
5. The patient should then be advised to empty the bladder, and to keep drinking as much as possible for the rest of the day. This will help to reduce the radiation dose to the bladder.

3.2.7 IMAGE LAYOUT

Right lateral skull	Left lateral skull
Anterior Right chest + shoulder and humerus	Anterior left chest + shoulder and humerus

	Posterior cervical dorsal spine
Anterior Pelvis	Posterior dorsal/lumber spine
Anterior Femora	Posterior Pelvis

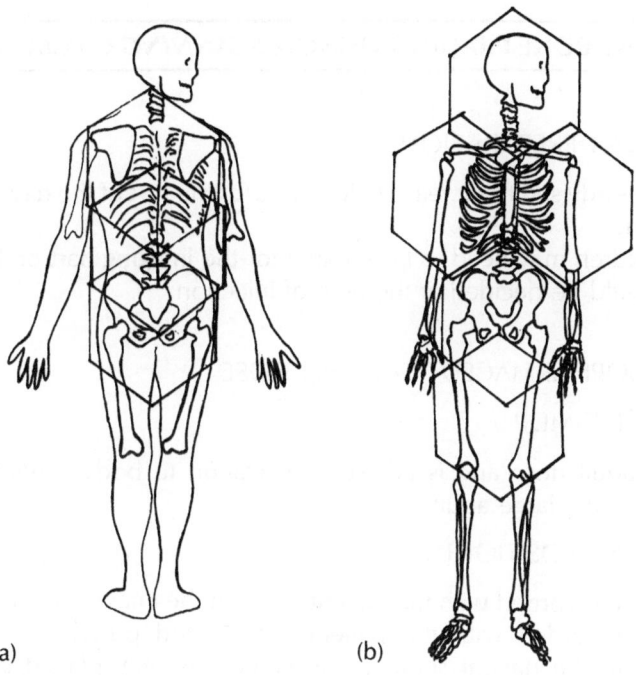

(a)   (b)

Fig. 3.1   Patient positioning for whole-body bone imaging: (a) posterior; (b) anterior.

3.3 ROUTINE BONE IMAGING USING A *SCANNING* GAMMA CAMERA

3.3.1 PATIENT PREPARATION

The patient is advised to increase fluid intake for the rest of the day following the injection.

Some children may need to be sedated for the imaging part of the study, and this should be decided at the time of injection.

3.3.2 RADIOPHARMACEUTICAL AND DOSE

550 MBq $^{99}Tc^m$-MDP

This is the adult dose and is adjusted in relation to body surface area in children and very large adults.

3.3.3 PATIENT POSITIONING

All images are recorded with the patient lying on the imaging table. Anterior images are recorded with the patient prone, and posterior images are recorded with the patient supine. The camera is only placed above the imaging table if the patient is unable to lie prone.

3.3.4 EQUIPMENT

The study is performed on a large-field-of-view scanning camera using a fishtail or high-resolution collimator.

3.3.5 COMPUTER

This is not normally used for whole-body bone scans with scanning cameras.

3.3.6 TECHNIQUE

1. Ensure patient has emptied bladder.
2. Ensure camera and film back are set (select whole body and dual intensity on the multiformatter).
3. Select scanning mode.
4. Position patient as in patient positioning. Ensure that there is a clear 1 cm gap between the base of the imaging table and the face of the collimator.

Position camera over patient's dorsal spine. Select the desired data density and determine the scanning speed.

5. Return camera to top of patient's head. Instruct patient to turn head to *right*.
6. Select the appropriate scan length.
7. Start scan.
8. Position patient for the anterior view with the head turned to *right*. Repeat steps 4–7 for this view. To calculate scan speed, position camera over the patient's sternum.

Note

The fishtail collimator is not recommended for routine multiple-view bone imaging (as with the general-purpose or high-resolution collimator) due to the distortion of the image caused by this collimator along one plane.

3.4 BONE FLOW STUDY

3.4.1 PATIENT PREPARATION

Nil. The patient should be advised to increase fluid intake for the rest of the day following the injection.

3.4.2 RADIOPHARMACEUTICAL AND DOSE

550 MBq ^{99}Tc^m-MDP

This is the adult dose and is adjusted in relation to body surface area in children and very large adults.

Patients having bone flow studies of the hands should be injected in a foot vein using the saline flush technique described in Section 7.6.6.

3.4.3 PATIENT POSITIONING

Most images are recorded with the patient lying on the imaging table. Anterior images are recorded with the patient supine, and the camera is positioned under the imaging table for posterior images.

For flow studies of the hands or feet, the patient is positioned sitting, with the hands or feet placed firmly on the camera. Ensure that the patient's head is not in the field of view of the camera.

3.4.4 EQUIPMENT

The study is normally performed on a wide-field-of-view gamma camera fitted with a high-resolution collimator. If this is not possible, then any other camera may be used, fitted with a general-purpose or high-resolution collimator.

3.4.5 COMPUTER

This is used, if available, for backing up the study. It is set up to record one frame per second for 40 s (dynamic phase) using a 64 × 64 byte matrix. The equilibrium-phase image is recorded on a 128 × 128 matrix (word or 12 bits) for 5 min or 500 000 counts, depending on which part of the body is being imaged.

3.4.6 TECHNIQUE

1. Attach two ^{57}Co marker sources to the appropriate area being imaged,

e.g. if imaging hips, attach them to each anterior superior iliac spine (ASIS), and mark their respective positions on the patient's skin, for later reference. In other bone flow studies, ensure that the markers are placed so as not to overlay the abnormal area being imaged.

2. Position camera over appropriate area of the patient.
3. Ensure computer is set.
4. Ensure camera and film back or multiformatter are set.
5. Give bolus injection of ^{99}Tc^m-MDP, starting camera and computer at moment of cuff release. If imaging the extremities, i.e. hands or feet, delay start of acquisition by 7–10 s.
6. Record image on camera for 40 s.
7. Remove the ^{57}Co markers.
8. At 1 min after injection, record the equilibrium image for 500 000– 750 000 counts (depending on which part of the body is being imaged) or for 5 min, if the count rate is low. A ^{57}Co marker spot is attached within the field of view of the collimator adjacent to the patient's *right* side.
9. Repeat step 8 for any other views requested.
10. The patient is then advised to increase fluid intake for the rest of the day and empty the bladder frequently. This will help to reduce the radiation dose to the bladder. Arrange an afternoon appointment for the patient for the delayed images at 3–4 h.
11. The images obtained later in the day are recorded in a 256 × 256 matrix for as long a time as practicable, usually for 20 min per view if a single view is requested. Multiple views, as is the case in studies of the knees or ankles, are recorded for 10 min per view.

3.4.7 IMAGE LAYOUT

0–40 s Dynamic Analogue	0–40 s Dynamic Digital
1 min Equilibrium Analogue	1 min Equilibrium Digital
Delayed Analogue	Delayed Digital

The combined analogue and digital images are only possible from some computerized gamma cameras.

3.5 SACROILIAC QUANTITATION STUDY

3.5.1 TECHNIQUE

1. Ensure patient has emptied the bladder before imaging.
2. Position patient supine with camera under the imaging table, centred over the sacrum.
3. The computer is set up to record one static image in a 128 × 128 matrix for 3 min, closing on overflow, and for this reason it is critical that the patient empties the bladder immediately prior to positioning.
4. Analogue images are not normally recorded. It should therefore be checked that the computer has recorded the study particularly where the computer system is being shared by two or more gamma cameras.

3.5.2 ANALYSIS

> **Note**
> There are several methods of analysing the study, and this is just one of them.

Recall the digital image and adjust the lower threshold until there is a clear black area between each sacroiliac joint (SIJ) and the sacrum. Using irregular regions of interest, carefully outline the right and left sacroiliac joints'. Then calculate

Background counts = Maximum pixel count in image
  × Lower threshold ÷ 100

This yields a background pixel count which represents the pixels with highest counts in the area between SIJs and sacrum, not an average counts per pixel for that region. Then calculate

$$\text{Normalized (right) SIJ counts} = \frac{\text{Counts in (right) SIJ region}}{\text{Number of pixels in region}}$$

$$\text{SIJ index (right)} = \frac{\text{Normalized (right) SIJ counts}}{\text{Background counts}} \times 100$$

Thus the SIJ index represents the ratio of the mean SIJ counts per pixel (for either right or left) to background pixel counts, multiplied by 100.

Each department should set up their own normal ranges.

CHAPTER FOUR

LIVER–SPLEEN STUDIES

Introduction

When microcolloidal particles are injected intravenously, they are removed from the circulation by the cells of the reticuloendothelial system by phagocytosis. In the normal individual about 80% of reticuloendothelial cells are in the liver, 5–10% in the spleen and the remainder are distributed throughout the red bone marrow. The distribution of these cells in the liver and spleen is fairly homogeneous and therefore an intravenous injection of a radiolabelled microcolloid in suspension will become evenly distributed throughout these organs.

The liver is a common site for primary and secondary metastatic disease and therefore the visualization of the internal structure of the liver is important. The radionuclide images provide valuable information about the shape, size and position of the liver and spleen. Abnormal tissue is detected by reduction in the radionuclide accumulation compared to the surrounding tissue. The reduction or 'cold spot' can also be caused by cysts and abscesses. Additional diagnostic information can be available if a dynamic flow study is obtained. Tumours show an early blush on the flow study and then become cold on the static images. Cysts on the other hand will remain cold during all phases of the study. Structures which lie over the liver will cause artefacts by attenuating the photons and give rise to image non-uniformity. This is a fairly common artefact caused by the right breast or a breast prosthesis and a repeat image with the breast elevated or prosthesis removed solves the problem.

With the introduction of ultrasound, the number of liver–spleen imaging studies, once forming a large part of the routine examinations in nuclear medicine, has now declined.

Administration of the same colloid preparations as liver–spleen imaging, but in much higher doses, allows the visualization of the bone marrow. The principal application of marrow imaging is the demonstration of the distribution and the extent of functioning bone marrow.

4.1 RADIOPHARMACEUTICALS

4.1.1 $^{99}Tc^m$-SULPHUR, $^{99}Tc^m$-TIN AND $^{99}Tc^m$-HSA COLLOIDS

All of the $^{99}Tc^m$-labelled colloid preparations listed above are suitable for most of the studies described in this chapter.

Note

Aseptic procedure   Switch on the laminar flow cabinet at least 30 min before starting.

Follow the manufacturer's instructions for the dispensing and use of the $^{99}Tc^m$-labelled colloid preparations.

---

1. Assay and label the vial with activity, volume, time, date, batch number and expiry time.
2. The appearance of the final preparation should be clear or slightly hazy. If a precipitate is visible, the preparation should *not* be used.
3. Use within the shelf-life of the preparation and store as indicated by the manufacturer.
4. Record the following in the radiopharmaceutical records book:
   (a) date
   (b) name of preparation
   (c) manufacturer's lot number
   (d) $^{99}Tc^m$ generator number
   (e) total activity in vial
   (f) volume
   (g) time of preparation
   (h) batch number

4.1.2 $^{99}Tc^m$-LABELLED DENATURED RBCs

Note

Aseptic procedure   Switch on the laminar flow cabinet at least 30 min before starting.

The water bath must also be switched on at least 60 min before starting, with at least 3 cm of water in it. The water-bath temperature should be set at 49°C.

---

1. The red blood cells are labelled with 370–550 MBq $^{99}Tc^m$ using a red-blood-cell labelling kit, as described in Chapter 7.

2. Transfer the vial containing the labelled red blood cells to a perforated lead pot in the water bath. Incubate at 49°C for 15 min. Every 5 min, invert the vial carefully (using tongs) several times to mix.
3. Measure the activity and label the vial with activity, volume, time, date, batch number, expiry time and *patient's name*.
4. Complete a sheet in the blood products record book including the following:
   (a) date
   (b) name of preparation
   (c) red-cell labelling kit lot number
   (d) $^{99}Tc^m$ generator number
   (e) total activity in vial (in MBq)
   (f) volume of final preparation
   (g) time
   (h) batch number
5. Attach a specimen label to the record sheet and one to the patient's request form.

4.2 LIVER–SPLEEN IMAGING

4.2.1 PATIENT PREPARATION

Nil.

4.2.2 RADIOPHARMACEUTICAL AND DOSE

150 MBq $^{99}Tc^m$-sulphur, $^{99}Tc^m$-tin colloid or $^{99}Tc^m$-HSA colloid

This is the adult dose, and should be corrected on the basis of body surface area in children and adults weighing 100 kg or more.

4.2.3 PATIENT POSITIONING

The study is normally performed with the patient standing. If the patient is unable to stand still for the duration of the study, the study can be performed with the patient sitting or lying.

If the study is being performed after a gallium study, the anterior view should be recorded with the patient lying and using the same gamma camera as was used for the gallium study, to enable superposition of the images, if necessary.

4.2.4 EQUIPMENT

A large-field-of-view camera is normally used, fitted with a general-purpose or high-resolution collimator. For children, the large-field camera may be used on 'Mag'.

4.2.5 COMPUTER

The computer is only necessary if liver–spleen subtraction is to be performed, usually following a gallium or labelled white-cell scan. Generally, only the anterior view is recorded, using the same sized matrix as that used for recording the gallium or white-cell study.

4.2.6 TECHNIQUE

In some patients, it may be necessary to perform a liver flow study, and for this the patient should be positioned supine with the camera centred over the liver, using marker sources, and the injection given as a bolus.

Following this, record images using the image layout for the first 5 min of the two-kidney renal study (see Section 1.2.7).

1. The radiopharmaceutical is injected intravenously and the patient then waits for a minimum of 15 min.

Note

If using $^{99}Tc^m$-tin colloid or $^{99}Tc^m$-HSA colloid, do not flush the syringe since there is a possibility that the blood may clot in the syringe.

---

2. Using the image layout below, record the following views: anterior, posterior, both laterals, anterior with costal margin marker (10 cm length of lead rubber, 1 cm wide, attached to the patient's right lower costal margin) and anterior with breasts elevated if necessary. All the images are recorded for 500 000 counts each or 5 min per view.

   In children, fewer counts are needed for the same count density – approximately 300 000.

4.2.7 IMAGE LAYOUT

Anterior	Posterior
Right lateral	Left lateral
Anterior + costal marker	Anterior, breasts elevated

4.3 BONE MARROW IMAGING

4.3.1 PATIENT PREPARATION

Nil.

4.3.2 RADIOPHARMACEUTICAL AND DOSE

350 MBq ^{99}Tc^m-sulphur, ^{99}Tc^m-tin or ^{99}Tc^m-HSA colloid

This is the standard adult dose, and is adjusted in children and large adults on the basis of body surface area.

4.3.3 PATIENT POSITIONING

The study is always performed with the patient lying on the imaging table. Anterior views are recorded with the patient lying supine and posterior views are recorded with the patient lying prone.

4.3.4 EQUIPMENT

A large-field-of-view gamma camera fitted with a general-purpose or high-resolution collimator is used.

4.3.5 COMPUTER

The study is always recorded on a computer for 5 min per view or using the time determined to record the anterior pelvis view (64 × 64 word matrix, or 128 × 128), *not* stopping on pixel overflow.

4.3.6 TECHNIQUE

1. Inject the patient intravenously with the measured dose of the radio-pharmaceutical. The patient then has to wait for a minimum of 15 min before imaging can commence.
2. Ensure patient has emptied the bladder immediately prior to imaging.
3. Position the patient as in Section 4.3.3, and begin by recording the anterior pelvis view for 300 000 counts (and note the time taken), or record each image for 5 min per view.
4. Record further views following the image layout below and using the same time as that taken for the first view (in step 3 above). Pieces of lead

rubber sheeting should be used for carefully masking out the liver–spleen activity, if necessary.

5. Following the bone marrow images, routine liver–spleen images should always be recorded.

4.3.7 IMAGE LAYOUT

Anterior Right shoulder and chest	Anterior Left shoulder and chest
Anterior Pelvis	Posterior Chest
Anterior Femora and knees	Posterior Pelvis
Lateral Skull	Anterior Liver + 10 cm lead marker
Anterior Liver	Posterior Liver
Right lateral Liver	Left lateral Liver

4.4 SPLEEN IMAGING WITH DENATURED RBCs

4.4.1 PATIENT PREPARATION

This study is usually performed following a standard liver–spleen study, if indicated. At least 48 h should be allowed for the decay of the $^{99}Tc^m$ colloid, injected for the liver–spleen study, before commencing this spleen imaging study.

The study may be combined with a splenic clearance study (see below).

4.4.2 RADIOPHARMACEUTICAL AND DOSE

70 MBq $^{99}Tc^m$-labelled autologous *denatured* RBCs.

4.4.3 PATIENT POSITIONING

This is the same as described for the liver–spleen study.

4.4.4 EQUIPMENT

The same gamma camera should be used as was used for the liver–spleen study (to allow for superposition of the images), fitted with a general-purpose or high-resolution collimator.

4.4.5 COMPUTER

All the images are recorded on a computer using a 128 × 128 matrix, for 300 000 counts each or 5 min per view, stopping on pixel overflow.

4.4.6 TECHNIQUE

> **Note**
> It is essential to check the label on the red-blood-cell vial before injecting the dose to ensure that the patient is reinjected with his or her own blood.

1. The denatured red blood cells are injected intravenously and the patient then waits for 45 min.
2. Following the image layout below, record each image for 300 000 counts or for 5 min per view.

4.4.7 IMAGE LAYOUT

Anterior	Posterior
Left anterior oblique	Left lateral
Anterior + costal marker	Left posterior oblique

4.5 SPLENIC CLEARANCE STUDY

The study is always combined with a splenic imaging study (see above).

4.5.1 PATIENT PREPARATION
Nil.

4.5:2 RADIOPHARMACEUTICAL AND DOSE
70 MBq ^{99}Tc^m-labelled autologous *denatured* RBCs

4.5.3 EQUIPMENT
A well-type scintillation gamma counter.

4.5.4 TECHNIQUE

> **Note**
> It is essential to check the label on the red-blood-cell vial before injecting the dose to ensure that the patient is reinjected with his or her own blood.

1. Inject the ^{99}Tc^m-labelled denatured red blood cells intravenously.
2. Take 4 ml blood samples at 3, 10, 20 and 30 min after injection, into EDTA tubes. Gently rotate each sample as soon as it is taken to prevent it from clotting.
3. At 45 min after injection, record images as for the splenic imaging study.

4.5.5 SAMPLE COUNTING AND CALCULATION

1. Haemolyse each sample by adding a knife point of saponin powder to each tube and gently mixing on the rotamixer for 5 min.
2. Transfer 2 ml aliquots from each sample to 10 ml counting tubes using separate pipettes for each sample, and count for 2 min each on a ^{99}Tc^m window using a gamma counter.
3. Plot the activity of the samples on linear graph paper, taking the 3 min sample as 100%.

4. Read off the following:
   (a) time taken to reach 50% of the activity at time 0 (normal range 9–18 min)
   (b) percentage of activity remaining at 20 min (normal range 17–46%)

4.6 PERITONEAL (LeVEEN) SHUNT STUDY

4.6.1 PATIENT PREPARATION

The patient should be instructed to void prior to examination.

4.6.2 RADIOPHARMACEUTICAL AND DOSE

70 MBq ^{99}Tc^m-sulphur, ^{99}Tc^m-tin colloid or ^{99}Tc^m-HSA colloid

4.6.3 PATIENT POSITIONING

The patient is positioned supine on the imaging table with the camera centred over the area of the LeVeen shunt. (The shunt should be palpable in the thoracic wall and on the lateral side of the neck.)

4.6.4 EQUIPMENT

A wide-field-of-view camera fitted with a general-purpose collimator is used.

4.6.5 COMPUTER

The computer is used to record dynamic images of one frame per second for 60 s in a 64 × 64 matrix, in byte mode. A further 2–3 images are recorded in a 128 × 128 matrix (word) for 5 min per view.

4.6.6 TECHNIQUE

1. Position patient as described under patient positioning.
2. Ensure camera and computer are set.
3. Pass a 20G needle through the abdominal wall until ascitic fluid is obtained.
4. Inject the radiopharmaceutical intraperitoneally, remove the needle and treat the puncture site by applying pressure.
5. Monitor the site using the persistence scope and start imaging as soon as activity appears in the lower portion of the tube.
6. Delayed views may need to be recorded up to 5 h after administering the dose if no activity is seen in the tube.

CHAPTER FIVE

GASTRIC STUDIES

> **Note**
> With some exceptions (see text for details), the patient should generally be fasted (clear fluids only) from midnight on the day of the study. Barium studies interfere, and double booking should always be checked for.

INTRODUCTION

Currently, hepatobiliary imaging may be the most sensitive and specific test for patients suffering from acute cholecystitis. The results are usually available within 1 h from the start of the study. Many ^{99}Tc^m-labelled derivatives of iminodiacetic acid are suitable for hepatobiliary imaging. Most of them are extracted by the liver and excreted into the bile in high concentrations.

Detection and quantitation of gastro-oesophageal reflux and oesophageal emptying are now standard investigations requiring a radioactive drink.

Biliary reflux studies may be carried out in patients who complain of abdominal discomfort following a fatty meal. They require the preparation of a fatty meal to which is added ^{111}In-DTPA. As with the dual phase gastric emptying studies, they require careful setting up of the imaging and data recording equipment in dual isotope imaging mode. Gastric emptying studies can be performed using a solid or a liquid phase marker, or both together. The rate of gastric emptying can be measured quantitatively, and is primarily of use in evaluating symptoms in postoperative gastric surgery patients. It is also used for monitoring the effects of drug therapy, as well as in untreated patients who complain of pain, heartburn and bloating. There is currently no other readily available quantitative technique for measuring gastric emptying.

^{99}Tc^m-Pertechnetate is secreted by the chief cells in gastric mucosa and therefore this agent can be used to localize Meckel's diverticulum. Most Meckel's diverticula which cause symptoms of gastrointestinal bleeding and pain contain gastric mucosa. This is a well-established test and is of particular value in children.

Location of GI bleeding using $^{99}Tc^m$-autologous red blood cells is now a routine technique. The technique is several times more sensitive than angiography. It is critical that the labelling efficiency of the red cells is greater than 98% otherwise the free pertechnetate will cause artefacts due to its secretion in the gastric mucosa and the kidneys. The only limitation is that the patient must be actively bleeding at the time of imaging for accurate localization, since the blood may move proximal to or distal from the bleeding site.

$^{99}Tc^m$-Pertechnetate is taken up by salivary and glandular tissue in a similar fashion to iodine. This uptake is utilized for imaging and functional evaluation of the salivary glands. Discharge of activity from the salivary glands can be produced by introducing a few drops of lemon juice in the patient's mouth.

The pulmonary inhalation study is effectively an extension of the oesophageal reflux study and is performed to document chronic aspiration. The test has become important in investigating infants with failure to thrive, recurrent vomiting and respiratory infections.

5.1 RADIOPHARMACEUTICALS

5.1.1 $^{99}Tc^m$-HIDA

There are several different derivatives of this compound available and the choice of use varies from one centre to another.

> **Note**
> *Aseptic procedure*   Switch on the laminar flow cabinet at least 30 min before starting.

1. Follow the manufacturer's instructions for the labelling, storage and use of the particular preparation utilized.
2. Measure the activity and label the vial with activity, volume, time, date, batch number and expiry time.
3. Use within the shelf-life specified by the manufacturer.
4. Record the following in the radiopharmaceutical records book:
   (a) date
   (b) name of preparation
   (c) manufacturer's lot number
   (d) $^{99}Tc^m$ generator number
   (e) total activity in vial
   (f) volume
   (g) time
   (h) batch number

5.1.2 $^{99}Tc^m$-LABELLED ACIDIFIED ORANGE DRINK

Formula

Analar HCl (0.1 N)	150 ml (A)
Orange squash	50 ml
Water,	to 100 ml (B)
Container	500 ml bottle in a lead container lined with a polythene bag

Procedure

1. Mix A and B to give a volume of 250 ml of acidified orange drink, place in bottle with lead shield and add 20 MBq $^{99}Tc^m$-sulphur or $^{99}Tc^m$-tin colloid.
2. Mix by swirling. Do *not* invert or shake.
3. Place the container in the lead pot.

4. Affix the label to the lid of the container and the lead pot.
5. A further 50 ml of water is supplied in a separate beaker to wash down the drink, giving a total volume of 300 ml ingested.

5.1.3 ^{111}In-LABELLED FATTY DRINK

Formula

Buildup (flavour of choice)	1 sachet
Casilan	1 tub (23 g)
Sugar	1 teaspoonful
Distilled water,	to 300 ml
Prosparol (well shaken)	25 ml
^{111}In-DTPA	20 MBq
Container	500 ml bottle in lead container lined with a polythene bag

Procedure

1. Empty the Buildup into a 500 ml calibrated bottle.
2. Add approximately 150 ml water and mix.
3. Add Casilan.
4. Mix together until smooth.
5. Make up to the 300 ml mark with distilled water and shake.
6. Add sugar and shake.
7. Add Prosparol and shake again for 1 min.
8. Add ^{111}In-DTPA and swirl to mix. Do *not* invert the bottle.
9. Place the bottle in the lead container.
10. Affix a label to the lid of the bottle and one to the lead container.

5.1.4 ^{99}Tc^m-LABELLED BRAN IN PORRIDGE

Formula

Bran	5 g
Instant porridge	50 g
Stannous chloride	10 mg
Sugar	1 teaspoonful
Hydrochloric acid (1 M)	*q.s.*
Milk	250 ml
^{99}Tc^m-pertechnetate	50 MBq
Distilled water	*q.s.*
Container	500 ml bottle in lead container lined with a polythene bag

Procedure for labelling bran

1. Weigh the bran into a 30 ml universal container.
2. Add 50 MBq ^{99}Tc^m-pertechnetate to a second universal container. Dilute to 15 ml with distilled water. Add two drops of 1 M hydrochloric acid (use a 1 ml syringe without a needle attached).
3. Add the resultant technetium solution to the bran.
4. Mix thoroughly using a whirlimixer for 2–3 min in the fume cupboard.
5. Weigh the stannous chloride into a fresh universal container, add two drops of 1 M hydrochloric acid and dilute to 10 ml with distilled water.
6. Add 2 ml of the stannous chloride solution to the bran mixture and mix ·thoroughly on a whirlimixer for 2–3 min.
7. Centrifuge at 1000 rpm for 5 min.
8. Pour the supernatant into a fresh universal container and add a similar quantity of fresh distilled water to the bran mixture.
9. Measure the activity in the bran container and the supernatant container and calculate the percentage of activity in the bran.
10. Thoroughly mix the bran mixture on the whirlimixer for 2–3 min. Centrifuge at 1000 rpm for 5 min and pour the supernatant into the universal container containing the first lot of supernatant. Add a similar quantity of distilled water to the bran mixture.
11. Repeat step 10.
12. After each washing, calculate the percentage of activity associated with the bran.
13. Repeat the washing until the percentage is constant to within 3%.

Preparing the instant porridge

1. Fifteen minutes before the meal is required, warm the milk to nearly boiling.
2. Add the milk to the instant porridge and mix thoroughly.
3. Add the ^{99}Tc^m-bran to the porridge and mix thoroughly so that the bran is mixed evenly through the porridge.
4. Place the bottle in the lead container.
5. Affix a label to the lid of the bottle and one to the lead container.

5.1.5 ^{111}-In-LABELLED MILK DRINK

Formula

Milk	250 ml
^{111}In-DTPA	20 MBq
Container	500 ml bottle in lead container lined with a polythene bag

Procedure

1. Put 250 ml of milk into the 500 ml container.
2. Add 20 MBq ^{111}In-DTPA.
3. Mix by swirling. Do *not* invert or shake.
4. Place the container in the lead pot.
5. Affix the label to the lid of the container and the lead pot.

5.2 HEPATOBILIARY IMAGING

The full study should be performed whenever possible. When the study is being performed for suspected *acute* cholecystitis, a limited study may be performed. A limited study comprises images recorded 30 min after injection; usually anterior and right lateral views are adequate.

5.2.1 PATIENT PREPARATION

The patient should be fasted overnight. If this is not possible, the patient should fast for 2 h before commencing the study.

5.2.2 RADIOPHARMACEUTICAL AND DOSE

200 MBq $^{99}Tc^m$-HIDA, injected IV

5.2.3 EQUIPMENT

A standard- or a wide-field-of-view gamma camera is used, fitted with a high-resolution or general-purpose collimator.

5.2.4 PATIENT POSITIONING

The study is performed with the patient lying supine on the imaging table, and the camera positioned over the right upper quadrant of the abdomen.

5.2.5 COMPUTER

The computer is not normally used but, if the facility is available, it can be used to back up the study.

5.2.6 TECHNIQUE

1. Set the clock for 30 min.
2. Ensure camera and film back or multiformatter are set.
3. Inject the dose intravenously.
4. At 2 min, record an image for 300 000 counts, with the intensity slightly reduced (1). Note the time required to record this image. If specified, a posterior and a right lateral view of the liver should be recorded at this stage.

5. Using the image layout below, record images (2–5) for the same time as taken for the 2 min image.
6. At 30 min, record a right lateral image (6) for the same time.
7. If the gall-bladder or gut are not visualized, repeat the anterior and right lateral images at 60 min, then hourly up to 4 h, or a dose of CCK (cholecystokinin) may be given intravenously followed by another dose of $^{99}Tc^m$-diethyl HIDA. Further images are recorded as in step 5.

5.2.7 IMAGE LAYOUT

1 2 min	2 5 min
3 10 min	4 20 min
5 30 min	6 Right lateral

5.3 GASTRIC (OESOPHAGEAL) REFLUX

5.3.1 PATIENT PREPARATION

The patient should be fasted (clear fluids only) from midnight on the day of the study. Barium studies interfere, and double booking should always be checked for.

5.3.2 RADIOPHARMACEUTICAL AND DOSE

20 MBq $^{99}Tc^m$-acidified orange drink

250 ml acidified $^{99}Tc^m$-acidified orange drink (20 MBq $^{99}Tc^m$-colloid) is needed, and a separate beaker containing 50 ml water.

5.3.3 EQUIPMENT

A wide-field-of-view gamma camera fitted with a general-purpose collimator or a standard-field camera fitted with a diverging collimator is used.

An abdominal binder is used to compress the patient's abdomen, and this should be checked, using a manometer, before the patient's arrival.

5.3.4 COMPUTER

The computer is set up to record multiple static images for 30 s duration each using a 64 × 64 word matrix.

5.3.5 TECHNIQUE

1. Administer the drink through a drinking straw with the patient sitting. After the drink, give the patient the 50 ml of water through the same straw.
2. Immediately, position the patient supine under the camera with the pressure cuff around the abdomen, but placed so that it is just below the ribs. Position the patient so that the persistence image of the stomach appears at the bottom of the screen.
3. Record images on the computer for 30 s per image at varying pressures starting at 0 mm of mercury and with incremental steps of 20 mm to a maximum of 100 mm of mercury. If the patient feels pain or discomfort at any pressure, record this on the form. If the discomfort is severe, the study should be terminated at that point.

5.3.6 ANALYSIS

The aim of the analysis is to display eight images corresponding to different cuff pressures.

The study is analysed by defining a region of interest over the oesophagus in each image to produce a pressure–activity trend curve which would display the degree of reflux, if reflux is occurring.

The amount of reflux can be quantitated by expressing the activity in the oesophagus as a percentage of the total activity in the stomach.

5.4 GASTRIC EMPTYING (DUAL LABEL)

5.4.1 PATIENT PREPARATION

The patient should be fasted (clear fluids only) from midnight on the day of the study. Barium studies interfere, and double booking should always be checked for.

5.4.2 RADIOPHARMACEUTICALS AND DOSE

Approximately 50 MBq ^{99}Tc^{m}-bran in porridge
20 MBq ^{111}In-milk drink

5.4.3 EQUIPMENT

A wide-field-of-view camera, fitted with the medium-energy collimator, is used. It should be equipped with appropriate electronics suitable for imaging dual isotopes simultaneously.

5.4.4 PATIENT POSITIONING

After ingesting the meal, the patient is positioned, as *quickly* as possible, in a 45° semi-recumbent position using a 'giant wedge' as back support (Fig. 5.1). The camera is positioned over the abdomen so that the stomach appears in the centre of the field of view as confirmed on the persistence scope.

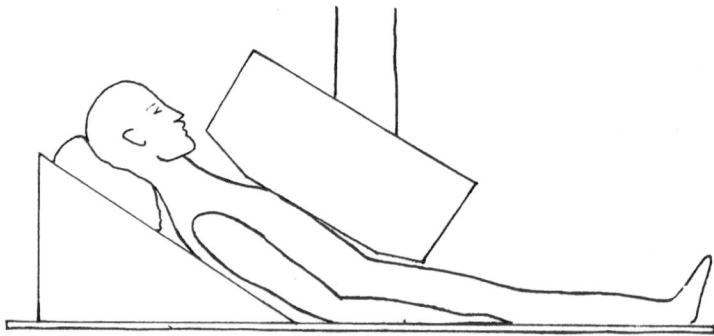

Fig. 5.1   Patient positioning for a gastric emptying study.

5.4.5 COMPUTER

The computer is set up to record in dual-isotope mode at a frame rate of one frame per minute using a 64 × 64 word matrix for 60 min (120 frames will be recorded; therefore, ensure that there is enough recording space on the system).

5.4.6 TECHNIQUE

1. Position low-activity $^{99}Tc^m$ and ^{111}In sources in front of the camera. Set the analyser windows to 12%.
2. Centre photopeaks using the multichannel analyser, ensuring that there is good separation between the peaks. The 173 keV peak of ^{111}In should be used.
3. Ensure that the camera is connected to the computer, including the Z_b lead. Set up the computer to record the study using the acquisition parameters described above.
4. Instruct the patient to consume the standard gastric emptying study meal by eating alternate mouthfuls of porridge and milk. The time taken to complete the meal should be noted on the patient's request form.
5. As soon as the patient has consumed the meal, position the patient immediately, as described earlier. The time taken to position the patient and start the acquisition should also be noted on the patient's request form.
6. There is no point in recording the analogue images.

5.4.7 ANALYSIS

The aim of the analysis is to produce time–activity curves for each radionuclide, by defining irregular regions of interest over the stomach. The curves should be corrected for crossover of $^{99}Tc^m$ into ^{111}In and vice versa, and the physical decay of $^{99}Tc^m$.

The half-times of clearance of each of the solid and liquid phases are calculated by analysing the exponential curves.

Note
The ROI over the stomach should be checked carefully, to ensure that the area being outlined is the stomach, particularly in post-surgical cases.

5.5 BILIARY (DUODENOGASTRIC) REFLUX

5.5.1 PATIENT PREPARATION

The patient should be fasted (clear fluids only) from midnight on the day of the study. Barium studies interfere, and double booking should always be checked for.

5.5.2 RADIOPHARMACEUTICALS AND DOSE

150 MBq ^{99}Tc^m-HIDA
20 MBq ^{111}In-fatty meal

5.5.3 EQUIPMENT

A wide-field-of-view camera, fitted with the medium-energy collimator, is used. It should be equipped with appropriate electronics suitable for imaging dual isotopes simultaneously.

5.5.4 PATIENT POSITIONING

The study is always performed with the patient lying supine on the imaging table.

5.5.5 COMPUTER

The computer is set up to record in dual-isotope mode at a frame rate of one frame per minute using a 64 × 64 word matrix for 60 min (120 frames will be recorded; therefore, ensure that there is enough recording space on the system).

5.5.6 TECHNIQUE

1. Position low-activity ^{99}Tc^m and ^{111}In sources in front of the camera. Set the analyser windows to 12%.
2. Centre photopeaks using the multichannel analyser, ensuring that there is good separation of the peaks. The 173 keV peak of ^{111}In should be used.
3. Ensure that the camera is connected to the computer, including the Z_b lead.
4. Inject the patient with the measured dose of ^{99}Tc^m-HIDA, intravenously.

5. Position the patient under the camera and visually monitor the right upper quadrant of the abdomen on the persistence scope until the gall-bladder and the common bile duct are full of activity. This usually occurs 15–30 min after the time of injection. For patients who have had cholecystectomy, proceed to the next step at 15 min after injection of the $^{99}Tc^m$-HIDA.
6. When the gall-bladder is full, ask the patient to sit up and give the ^{111}In-fatty drink through a flexistraw, to be drunk within 5 min or less. Note the time taken by the patient to consume the drink.

   Set up to record in dual-isotope mode at a frame rate of one frame per minute in matrix 4 (64 × 64 word) for 60 min.
7. Position the patient as described above and start the data acquisition on the system being used.
8. Select the dual-display option on the camera console and record images on film every 5 min for 60 s each for the duration of the study, i.e. 1 h.

5.5.7 IMAGE LAYOUT

^{111}In $^{99}Tc^m$ 0 min	^{111}In $^{99}Tc^m$ 5 min
^{111}In $^{99}Tc^m$ 10 min	^{111}In $^{99}Tc^m$ 15 min
^{111}In $^{99}Tc^m$ 20 min	^{111}In $^{99}Tc^m$ 25 min
^{111}In $^{99}Tc^m$ 30 min	^{111}In $^{99}Tc^m$ 35 min
^{111}In $^{99}Tc^m$ 40 min	^{111}In $^{99}Tc^m$ 45 min
^{111}In $^{99}Tc^m$ 50 min	^{111}In $^{99}Tc^m$ 60 min

5.5.8 ANALYSIS

The studies are analysed as follows:

1. Select the ^{111}In image and, using irregular regions of interest, outline the stomach.
2. Select the ^{99}Tc^m-HIDA image and outline the liver, but exclude the gall-bladder.
3. Generate time–activity curves for both regions on both images.
4. In order to correct for crossover of ^{111}In counts in the ^{99}Tc^m window, the stomach counts in the ^{111}In window should be multiplied by the crossover correction factor. It is recommended that each system be calibrated by the user centre to determine this factor.

The aim of the analysis is to generate these curves to illustrate whether there is any indication of reflux.

The half-time of the ^{111}In meal clearance from the stomach is calculated by fitting an exponential to the stomach ROI curve.

5.6 OESOPHAGEAL CLEARANCE

5.6.1 PATIENT PREPARATION

The patient must have fasted for at least 2 h prior to the study.

5.6.2 RADIOPHARMACEUTICAL AND DOSE

15 ml water and 10 MBq $^{99}Tc^m$-colloid

15 ml of tap water is dispensed into a universal container in a lead pot and 10 MBq of $^{99}Tc^m$-colloid is added. A second universal container containing only tap water is also needed.

5.6.3 EQUIPMENT

A large-field-of-view camera is preferred. Alternatively, a standard-field-of-view camera fitted with a diverging collimator can also be used.

5.6.4 PATIENT POSITIONING

The study is performed with the patient upright and/or supine.

5.6.5 COMPUTER

The computer is set up to record one frame per second for 15 s, then at one frame every 15 s in a 64 × 64 matrix for 40 frames (10 min).

5.6.6 TECHNIQUE

1. Position the patient in front of or under the camera, with the camera centred over the chest so that the area between the suprasternal notch and the umbilicus is within the field of view. Explain the technique to the patient.
2. Using the universal container containing the tap water, give the patient a practice run swallowing the water in one go and then swallowing at 15 s intervals (and not at any other times) up to 5 min.
3. Position the container with activity by the patient, with a flexistraw in the mouth. Instruct the patient to drink the entire dose in one swallow. Begin the computer acquisition simultaneously.
4. At 15 s tell the patient to swallow. Thereafter prompt the patient to swallow every 15 s and to avoid doing so at other times.

5.6.7 ANALYSIS

1. Select the first frame of the study.
2. Add the first 15 images of the study to produce a composite image over the first phase of the study.
3. Using this image, outline the activity in the oesophagus using a rectangular region of interest.
4. Note the total activity in the ROI (*TOT*).
5. Calculate the clearance at each time C as

$$\text{Clearance (\%)} = \frac{\text{Counts at time } C}{TOT} \times 100$$

6. Plot the curve of percentage clearance against time.

5.7 MECKEL'S DIVERTICULUM IMAGING

5.7.1 PATIENT PREPARATION

The study is always performed with the patient fasting.

5.7.2 RADIOPHARMACEUTICAL AND DOSE

200 MBq $^{99}Tc^m$-pertechnetate injected IV

This is the adult dose and is reduced in children on the basis of their body surface area.

5.7.3 EQUIPMENT

A large-field-of-view gamma camera fitted with a general-purpose or high-resolution collimator is used. If a standard-field camera is to be used, the diverging collimator should be fitted for large adults.

5.7.4 PATIENT POSITIONING

The patient is positioned supine on the imaging table with the camera positioned over the abdomen so that the whole abdomen from the bladder to the xiphisternum is in the field of view (Fig. 5.2).

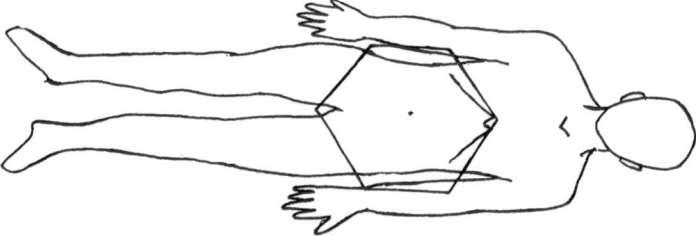

Fig. 5.2   Patient positioning for a Meckel's diverticulum study.

5.7.5 COMPUTER

This is not normally used, but, if the facility is available, it can be used for backing up the study. It should be set up as the study progresses using a 128 × 128 word matrix and recording for the same length of time as the analogue images. Alternatively, it could be set up to record 30 frames at one frame per minute in a 64 × 64 word matrix.

5.7.6 TECHNIQUE

1. Ensure computer is set, if using one.
2. Set clock for 30 min.
3. Ensure camera and film back or multiformatter are set.
4. Give bolus injection of $^{99}Tc^m$-pertechnetate, starting camera (and computer) at moment of cuff release.
5. Record first image on camera for 30 s (1).
6. At 1 min after injection, record an image for 400 000 counts (2). Note the time taken for this image on the patient's request form for later reference in case a delayed image needs to be recorded.
7. Following the image layout below, record images at 5, 10, 20 and 30 min for the same length of time as taken for the 1 min image.

Further images may need to be recorded. The physician on duty usually decides this.

5.7.7. IMAGE LAYOUT

0–30 s	1 min
5 min	10 min
20 min	30 min

5.8 LOCALIZATION OF GASTROINTESTINAL BLEEDING WITH ^{99}Tc^m-RBCs

5.8.1 PATIENT PREPARATION

This study is usually only performed on patients in whom there is a strong clinical suspicion of gastrointestinal bleeding.

No formal preparation is needed, but it may be helpful to pass a nasogastric tube (if not already done), and maintain suction. This is necessary so that any free pertechnetate may be aspirated as it is secreted in the stomach.

5.8.2 RADIOPHARMACEUTICAL AND DOSE

750 MBq autologous ^{99}Tc^m-RBC

> **Note**
> The red-cell labelling efficiency should be checked to ensure that there is no free pertechnetate. If there is any, then the labelled cells should be washed using 0.9% w/v sodium chloride for injections.

5.8.3 PATIENT POSITIONING

The study is performed with the patient supine. Normally only anterior views are recorded, but occasionally lateral and oblique views may need to be recorded.

5.8.4 EQUIPMENT

The study is performed using a large-field-of-view gamma camera, fitted with a general-purpose or high-resolution collimator.

5.8.5 COMPUTER

This is not normally used, but, if available, it can be used for backing up the study. It should be set up as the study progresses using a 128 $\times$ 128 word matrix and recording for the same length of time as the analogue images. Alternatively, it could be set up to record 30 frames at one frame per minute in a 64 $\times$ 64 word matrix.

5.8.6 TECHNIQUE

1. Using ^{57}Co marker sources, ensure that the whole abdomen from the

diaphragm to the ischium is in the field of view of the camera.
2. Ensure computer is set, if using one.
3. Set clock for 30 min.
4. Ensure camera and film back or multiformatter are set.
5. Inject the ^{99}Tc^m-RBC using the saline flush technique of bolus administraton (see Section 7.6.6), starting camera (and computer) at moment of cuff release.
6. Record the first image on camera for 30 s (1).
7. At 1 min after injection, record an image for 1 000 000 counts (2), ensuring that the heart is not in the field of view. Note the time taken for this image on the patient's request form for later reference.
8. Record further images every 5 min up to 30 min for the same length of time as taken to record the 1 min image.
9. Later images are recorded every 15 min for the next 6 h for the same length of time, but corrected for decay of ^{99}Tc^m.

5.8.7 IMAGE LAYOUT

1 0–30 s	2 1 min
3 5 min	4 10 min
5 15 min	6 20 min
25 min	30 min

5.9 SALIVARY GLAND IMAGING (STATIC)

5.9.1 PATIENT PREPARATION

No patient preparation is needed for this study.

5.9.2 RADIOPHARMACEUTICAL AND DOSE

185 MBq ^{99}Tc^m-pertechnetate injected IV

5.9.3 EQUIPMENT

A standard-field-of-view gamma camera is used, fitted with a high-resolution collimator. If a wide-field camera is used, the camera should be set to 'Mag'. The images may also be recorded in zoomed mode on the data system.

5.9.4 PATIENT POSITIONING

The patient is positioned supine on the imaging table.

5.9.5 COMPUTER

Each image is recorded on a computer, if available, using a 128 × 128 or a 256 × 256 matrix recording for 5 min per view.

5.9.6 TECHNIQUE

1. Inject the patient intravenously with the measured dose of ^{99}Tc^m-pertechnetate.
2. The patient then waits for 30 min.
3. At 30 min after injection, position the patient under the camera, and record an anterior and both lateral views for 5 min each. When recording the anterior view, ensure that the neck is well extended.
4. If there is any possibility of a lesion in a salivary gland, a magnified view may be needed. A pinhole or a converging collimator should be used for recording this.

5.9.7 IMAGE LAYOUT

Anterior	
Right lateral	Left lateral

5.10 SALIVARY GLAND IMAGING (DYNAMIC)

5.10.1 PATIENT PREPARATION

None.

5.10.2 RADIOPHARMACEUTICAL AND DOSE

185 MBq ^{99}Tc^{m}-pertechnetate injected IV

A small quantity (1 ml) of fresh lemon juice or concentrated lemon squash is also necessary.

5.10.3 PATIENT POSITIONING

The patient is positioned supine with a pillow under the shoulders so that the neck is well extended.

5.10.4 EQUIPMENT

A standard-field-of-view gamma camera is used, fitted with a general-purpose collimator. If a wide-field gamma camera is to be used, it should be set to 'Mag'.

5.10.5 COMPUTER

The computer is set up to record one frame per minute using a 64 × 64 word matrix for 15 min.

5.10.6 TECHNIQUE

1. Position the patient as described above. A head clamp may be used to ensure that the patient does not move. Using ^{57}Co marker sources, ensure that the area from the nasion to the suprasternal notch is in the field of view.
2. Ensure computer is set.
3. Set clock for 15 min.
4. Ensure camera and film back or multiformatter are set.
5. Inject the patient intravenously with the measured dose of ^{99}Tc^{m}-pertechnetate, starting camera and computer at moment of injection.
6. Record images for 1 min duration each at 2, 5, 7, 9, 12 and 15 min as in

image layout below. At 10 min after starting acquisition, give the patient a few drops of concentrated lemon squash or fresh lemon juice using a dropper or a syringe. This must be carried out without moving the patient.

7. If static views are required, these should be recorded at 30 min after injection as described in the next section.

5.10.7 IMAGE LAYOUT

2 min	5 min
7 min	9 min
12 min	15 min

5.10.8 ANALYSIS

The analysis is carried out by summing all the images and outlining the four salivary glands individually using irregular regions of interest.

Time–activity curves are plotted (Fig. 5.3) and two sets of hard-copy images are recorded so that one copy may be sent out with the patient's scan report. The curves should show normal instantaneous discharge of activity from the salivary glands soon after the lemon juice is given to the patient.

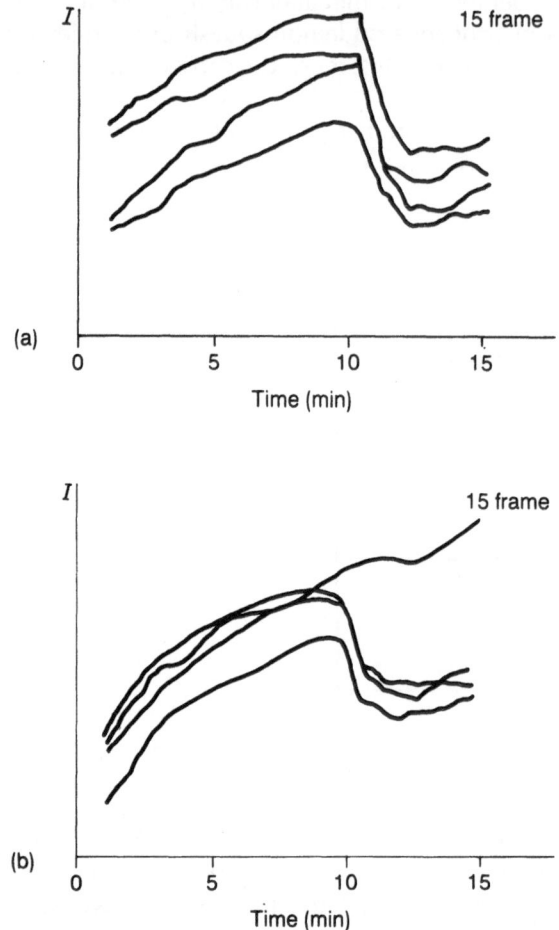

Fig. 5.3 Time–activity curves from a dynamic salivary gland study: (a) normal study, (b) obstructed salivary gland.

CHAPTER SIX

LUNG IMAGING STUDIES

INTRODUCTION

Perfusion lung imaging has been a well-established screening test for the detection of pulmonary embolus for several decades. Until a few years ago the perfusion lung scan was reviewed in conjunction with the patient's current chest X-ray to establish the diagnosis of PE. However, with the availability of radioactive gases and radioaerosol systems, the combined ventilation and perfusion lung scan is now routinely used to accurately diagnose PE. Quantitation of regional lung ventilation and perfusion is also possible if the images are recorded on a computer system.

Lung perfusion imaging is generally very safe, but patients with known pulmonary hypertension have a small risk of developing right heart failure, and therefore, patients with pulmonary hypertension should have their condition made known to the nuclear medicine personnel before the examination commences.

Macroaggregates of human serum albumin (MAA) labelled with $^{99}Tc^m$ are generally used for lung perfusion imaging because they are cheaper than microspheres to manufacture. Microspheres should be used in patients with right-to-left shunt in order to minimize the dangers of embolization since the particle size is smaller in range compared to macroaggregates. It is important that the vial containing the labelled MAA or microspheres is vigorously shaken before drawing up the dose, otherwise clumping together of the particles occurs and will consequently be reflected as image artefacts on the perfusion images.

Lung ventilation images can be obtained using $^{81}Kr^m$ gas which is generator-produced and has a half-life of 13 s with 0.19 MeV emission. Because of the short half-life there are no problems with disposal. The short half-life of the parent ^{81}Rb (4.7 h) means that difficulties are experienced in obtaining the generator by users on sites distant from the supplier since the generator must be used on the day of preparation. The use of $^{81}Kr^m$ for emergency lung ventilation imaging is therefore limited.

The disadvantages of availability of $^{81}Kr^m$ can be overcome by the use of

^{99}Tc^m aerosol or ^{133}Xe gas, which are readily available. ^{133}Xe has a longer half-life of 5.3 d and a principal energy of 0.80 MeV. The long half-life poses disposal problems although commercial traps are now available.

6.1 RADIOPHARMACEUTICALS

6.1.1 ^{99}Tc^m-MAA

> **Note**
> *Aseptic procedure*   Switch on the laminar flow cabinet at least 30 min before starting.

1. Collect the following:
   (a) one vial of MAA kit
   (b) one lead pot
   (c) one 10 ml syringe with 21G (green) needle
   (d) ^{99}Tc^m-pertechnetate
   (e) vial of 0.9% w/v sodium chloride for injections
   (f) one swab (isopropyl alcohol or chlorhexidine)
2. Remove the central metal disc from the MAA labelling vial.
3. Swab the rubber closures of the labelling, pertechnetate and saline vials.
4. Place the labelling vial in the lead pot.
5. Transfer the manufacturer's recommended volume and activity of pertechnetate to the MAA labelling vial. Withdraw an equal volume of gas from the vial. Shake the vial.
6. Measure the activity and label the vial with activity, volume, time, date, batch number and expiry time.
7. Follow the manufacturer's instructions on storage and use within the recommended shelf-life.
8. Record the following in the radiopharmaceutical records book
   (a) date
   (b) name of preparation
   (c) manufacturer's lot number
   (d) ^{99}Tc^m generator number
   (e) total activity in vial
   (f) volume
   (g) time
   (h) batch number

6.1.2 ^{81}Kr^m GAS GENERATOR

Setting up the generator

Full instructions for setting up the generator are usually enclosed in the generator. It is necessary to have a certain amount of secondary lead shielding around the generator container.

Connect the humidifier between the compressed air cylinder and the generator. Fill the humidifier reservoir with distilled water. Normal saline solution should *not* be used instead of water as it has been found to cause the breakthrough of the parent ^{81}Rb.

Checking the generator

After setting up the generator, turn on the air supply to 5 pounds per square inch, turn on the fans, peak the camera on ^{81}Kr^{m} and check that the count rate from the delivery end of the tube is at least 100 000 counts per minute.

6.2 PERFUSION LUNG IMAGING

6.2.1 PATIENT PREPARATION

None.

6.2.2 RADIOPHARMACEUTICAL AND DOSE

^{99}Tc^m-MAA

A fixed volume is used as a standard dose. A standard adult dose should contain approximately 400 000 particles and have an activity of 70–200 MBq. This dose is reduced in children in accordance with their body surface area.

The volume may vary from one kit manufacturer to another, and the manufacturer's instructions should be read carefully.

In patients who are suspected of having a right-to-left cardiac shunt or known pulmonary hypertension, the dose should be reduced by 50% in terms of the volume injected.

The vial of labelled MAA should be stored at 2–8°C.

6.2.3 PATIENT POSITIONING

The study is usually performed with the patient standing or sitting against the camera. Patients who are not able to stand or sit are imaged lying supine on the imaging table and the camera or patient position adjusted to record each appropriate view.

6.2.4 COMPUTER

A computer is only necessary if divided pulmonary function is to be calculated. Only anterior and posterior views are required and should be recorded using a 128 × 128 word matrix.

6.2.5 TECHNIQUE

1. The injection technique is as follows:
   (a) Shake the vial before drawing up the dose. The dose should not be drawn up and left in the syringe for any length of time as the particles tend to stick to the walls of the syringe. Also avoid injecting through any plastic tubing such as drip lines.

(b) Use a 21G needle to draw up and inject the dose.

(c) The patient should be positioned supine for the injection to ensure even distribution of the particles throughout the two lung fields.

(d) Invert the syringe containing the measured dose of the MAA several times to mix. Insert the needle into a suitable antecubital vein, draw back blood into the dead space of the syringe only to check that the venepuncture is successful and inject slowly with the patient breathing normally.

Note

Do not draw blood back into the syringe before injecting the MAA as there is a possibility of the MAA clumping.

(e) Flush the syringe three times.

2. Imaging should commence as soon as possible after injection. Following the image layout below, record anterior, posterior, both laterals and both posterior oblique views for 500 000 counts each or for 5 min each if the count rate is too low.

3. A current chest radiograph is always required for reporting. If a current chest radiograph has not been done, one should be requested following the scan.

6.2.6 IMAGE LAYOUT

Anterior	Posterior
Left posterior oblique	Right posterior oblique
Left lateral	Right lateral

Note that this image layout is for patients having perfusion studies only. See below for image layout for patients having perfusion and ventilation studies.

6.3 ^{81}Kr^m VENTILATION LUNG IMAGING

6.3.1 PATIENT PREPARATION

The patient will usually have a perfusion lung study performed first.

6.3.2 RADIOPHARMACEUTICALS AND DOSE

^{81}Kr^m from a ^{81}Rb generator

6.3.3 EQUIPMENT

A large-field-of-view gamma camera is used, fitted with a medium-energy collimator. Fans should be used to disperse the gas, and should be positioned so that the gas is blown away from the field of view of the camera. Care should be taken about the direction of the draught, as some camera detectors have in-built fans to keep the detector assembly cool by drawing air in from the outside, which would give rise to excessive background on the images if the ^{81}Kr^m gets inside the detector.

6.3.4 PATIENT POSITIONING

The patient is normally positioned standing against the camera. If the patient is unable to do so, then the images may be recorded with the patient sitting or lying.

6.3.5 COMPUTER

A computer is only necessary for calculating divided pulmonary function. It may also be used for subtracting the perfusion images from the ventilation images if desired. The matching pairs of images should be recorded for the same length of time if subtraction is to be performed. In all cases record using a 128 × 128 word matrix.

6.3.6 TECHNIQUE

1. Ensure fans are positioned to blow in the correct direction. Check that the camera, film back or multiformatter are set.
2. Position patient with face-mask attached to generator outlet tubing.
3. Turn on the air supply at a pressure of 5 pounds per square inch.

4. Position patient so that the face-mask is out of the field of view of the camera.
5. Begin by recording the posterior view for 500 000 counts and note the time taken. Record any other views requested for the same length of time as taken for this posterior view.

Note

If the ^{81}Kr^m activity is high, then the anterior, posterior and both oblique ventilation views should be recorded routinely. If the ^{81}Kr^m activity is low, only selected ventilation views need be recorded.

6.3.7 IMAGE LAYOUT

This is shown below, assuming all ventilation images are requested. Lateral ventilation images are not useful due to the shine-through from the opposite lung.

Anterior Perfusion	Anterior Ventilation
Posterior Perfusion	Posterior Ventilation
Right posterior oblique Perfusion	Right posterior oblique Ventilation
Left posterior oblique Perfusion	Left posterior oblique Ventilation
Left lateral Perfusion	
Right lateral Perfusion	

6.4 ^{99}Tc^m-DTPA AEROSOL VENTILATION LUNG IMAGING

6.4.1 PATIENT PREPARATION

Nil.

6.4.2 RADIOPHARMACEUTICAL AND DOSE

^{99}Tc^m-DTPA (370 MBq/ml)

6.4.3 EQUIPMENT

A large-field-of-view gamma camera is used fitted with a general-purpose or high-resolution collimator.

A commercially available radioaerosol inhalation apparatus is used, together with the following, which are not usually supplied with the apparatus:

1. Compressed air cylinder with a single airflow meter attached to it (oxygen is not recommended, as adverse reactions may occur following prolonged breathing with oxygen).
2. Nose clip.
3. Suitable trolley for the nebulizer to stand on.

6.4.4 PATIENT POSITIONING

The study is usually performed with the patient standing or sitting against the camera. Patients who are not able to stand or sit are imaged lying supine on the imaging table and the camera or patient position adjusted to record each appropriate view.

6.4.5 COMPUTER

The computer may be used for subtracting the perfusion images from the ventilation images or simply for backing up the images if the facility is available. The images should be recorded for the same length of time as the analogue images, using a 128 × 128 matrix.

6.4.6 TECHNIQUE

1. Position the patient in a comfortable recumbent/semi-recumbent position. This aids even distribution throughout the lungs, preventing sedimenta-

tion into the bases. Ideally ventilate the patient in a separate room to avoid possible contamination of the inner electronics of the gamma camera head by possible leakage of the aerosol.

2. Assemble the ventilation system and check that all the connections are secure. If in doubt, then apply insulation tape around each joint to prevent leaks. Prime the nebulizer with the recommended volume and activity of ^{99}Tc^m-DTPA (e.g. 925 MBq in 2.5 ml). Top up this amount by the recommended volume for each additional patient (e.g. 370 MBq in 1 ml).

3. Instruct the patient as to what is required of the patient during the ventilation procedure.
   (a) Ensure that the mouthpiece is held firmly and sealed tightly with the lips.
   (b) The patient should breath normally.
   (c) The patient must have a mouthwash on completion of the ventilation.

4. Place the nose clip on the patient's nose and ask the patient to breath through the mouthpiece as normally as possible. Ensure the patient is as comfortable as possible and turn on the air supply to 10 l/min pressure.

5. At 2 min after starting, turn off the air supply and let the patient carry on breathing through the apparatus for a further 15 s.

6. Remove the nose clip and give the patient a mouthwash.

7. Record a minimum of posterior and two posterior oblique views as soon as possible after ventilation for 500 000 counts each or for 5 min each.

8. Following the ventilation study, the patient should be left for between 1 and 1.5 h before perfusion studies are attempted. Patients in renal failure may have to be left for 6 h before perfusion imaging in order for the background activity to diminish.

6.5 VENTILATION LUNG IMAGING USING ^{133}Xe

6.5.1 PATIENT PREPARATION

Nil.

6.5.2 RADIOPHARMACEUTICAL AND DOSE

370 MBq ^{133}Xe in 6 l of air

6.5.3 EQUIPMENT

A large-field-of-view gamma camera is used, fitted with a general-purpose collimator. A commercially available ^{133}Xe rebreathing system is also needed.

6.5.4 PATIENT POSITIONING

The study is performed with the patient sitting with the back against the gamma camera, as only the posterior view is recorded.

6.5.5 COMPUTER

If the facility is available, record each image on the computer for the same length of time or the same number of counts as the analogue images, using the 128 × 128 matrix.

6.5.6 TECHNIQUE

1. Ensure camera, multiformatter and computer are set. Select 20% window and centre it on the 81 keV peak of ^{133}Xe.
2. Position the patient to include whole of the lung fields.
3. Explain the procedure to the patient. Attach the face-mask and have a practice run. When you are happy that the patient understands what is expected, inject the ^{133}Xe into the inlet airway and tell the patient to inhale deeply and hold the breath for as long as possible. Start the acquisition on the camera and computer and record the wash-in image for the duration of the breath hold. A minimum of 15 s should be recorded.
4. Let the patient breath normally into the system and record the equilibrium image on film as well as the computer for 300 000 counts. The camera intensity should be decreased for this image.

5. Switch on the ^{133}Xe machine to washout cycle, let the patient breathe normally and record three more images on film and computer from 0 to 1 min, 1 to 3 min and 3 to 6 min. The camera intensity will need to be increased for recording these images.

   (The ^{133}Xe is washed out of the machine into a special trap where it is absorbed onto activated charcoal. A mixture of oxygen and carbon dioxide is used to wash out the xenon from the trap.)

6. Process the film and check the images before proceeding to routine lung perfusion imaging.

6.5.7 IMAGE LAYOUT

Wash in + breath hold	Equilibrium
Washout 0–1 min	Washout 1–3 min
Washout 3–6 min	

CHAPTER SEVEN

CARDIAC STUDIES

INTRODUCTION

Thallium stress and redistribution imaging is performed for the detection and evaluation of known or suspected coronary artery disease (CAD) and for the follow-up of medical or surgical therapy in this group of patients.

Thallium acts as a potassium analogue and its distribution parallels blood flow and tissue viability. A resting thallium study has limited sensitivity for detecting ischaemic myocardium although it is very sensitive in detecting myocardial scarring and acute infarction. The sensitivity of thallium imaging for detecting myocardial ischaemia is greatly increased by injecting the thallium during peak exercise and imaging the patient as soon as possible thereafter. Patients are then reimaged after a 3 h delay to help separate ischaemic (changing or reperfusing) areas from myocardial scars (no change).

Many centres are now using rotating gamma camera tomography instead of planar imaging for thallium scintigraphy. There are now several $^{99}Tc^m$-labelled isonitrile complexes undergoing clinical trials for myocardial imaging. One of the most promising of these appears to be $^{99}Tc^m$-methoxyisobutylisonitrile (MIBI). This agent can be injected in comparatively higher doses than thallium and far better resolution is achieved due to the imaging characteristics of $^{99}Tc^m$. It also produces excellent tomographic images because of the improved statistics due to the increased photon flux, which also results in reduction in imaging times.

$^{99}Tc^m$-Pyrophosphate (PYP) is used for the detection of acute myocardial infarction. It is the presence of the influx of calcium ions into acutely necrotic tissue, with the formation of ultramicroscopic crystals resembling hydroxyapatite, which is thought to account for the uptake of PYP. The imaging can be carried out on the ward using a mobile gamma camera.

A left-to-right intracardiac shunt can be detected and quantified fairly accurately by recording a dynamic study following a good intravenous bolus injection of a radionuclide. In the presence of a shunt, early tracer recirculation occurs through the lungs, distorting the normal shape of the time–activity curve of the region of interest defined over the lung. This technique can be used to evaluate children or adults with suspected congenital or acquired heart disease for the presence of left-to-right intracardiac shunt. The procedure requires about 5 min of patient time. Patients with known left-to-right shunts such as atrial septal defects (ASD) or ventricular septal defects (VSD) can be studied in a serial manner to see, for example, the effect of surgical closure, or if spontaneous closure of the shunt is occurring.

A good bolus injection technique is the most important consideration since analysis of the data from a fragmented bolus injection will give a false positive study or an over-estimation of the degree of shunting.

Right-to-left shunts can be detected and accurately quantified by injecting $^{99}Tc^m$-labelled microspheres intravenously. If a right-to-left shunt is present, systemic and pulmonary deposition of the microspheres occurs. The test is often used in patients following surgical shunt closures. Provided that care is taken to limit the number of microspheres injected, there is no hazard to the patient from this procedure.

One of the most non-invasive techniques for the measurement of the ejection fraction is by utilizing multiple gated images and calculating the ejection fraction based on a time–activity curve over the cardiac cycle. Abnormalities of regional wall motion can be analysed by the change in the configuration of the cardiac blood pool. A non-invasive method of determining ejection fraction is useful in both the initial evaluation of patients with suspected cardiac disease and, for example, in following progress of treatment in patients who may be undergoing therapy with drugs which may be cardiotoxic. Using a suitable blood pool agent, ideally $^{99}Tc^m$-labelled autologous RBCs, studies can be repeated rapidly and serial ejection fraction measurements can be made at rest and with exercise intervention.

The technique does not require any patient preparation, although due to the fact that the patients being studied may have life-threatening cardiac problems, emergency equipment and appropriate medical staff should be available during the study.

7.1 RADIOPHARMACEUTICALS

7.1.1 ^{201}Tl-THALLOUS CHLORIDE

This is received ready for use, and the only procedure necessary is to check the total activity in the vial against the label.

7.1.2 ^{99}Tc^m-PYROPHOSPHATE

Note

Aseptic procedure   Switch on the laminar flow cabinet at least 30 min before starting. Swab with 0.5% chlorhexidine in 70% spirit.

---

1. Collect the following:
   (a) vial of PYP (pyrophosphate) kit
   (b) one lead pot
   (c) one 5 ml syringe with 21G (green) needle
   (d) ^{99}Tc^m-pertechnetate
   (e) one swab (isopropyl alcohol or chlorhexidine)
2. Remove the central metal disc from the pyrophosphate labelling vial.
3. Swab the rubber closures of the labelling and pertechnetate vials.
4. Place the labelling vial in the lead pot.
5. Transfer the volume and activity of ^{99}Tc^m-pertechnetate, as recommended by the manufacturer, into the labelling vial. Withdraw an equal volume of gas from the vial.
6. Shake for 1 min.
7. Assay and label the vial with activity, volume, time, date, batch number and expiry time.
8. Use within the recommended shelf-life.
9. Record the following in the radiopharmaceutical records book:
   (a) date
   (b) name of preparation
   (c) manufacturer's lot number
   (d) ^{99}Tc^m generator number
   (e) total activity in vial
   (f) volume
   (g) time
   (h) batch number

7.1.3 $^{99}Tc^m$-RBCs (KIT METHOD)

Note

Aseptic procedure Switch on the microbiological safety cabinet at least 5 min before starting

---

1. Collect the following:
   (a) red-blood-cell labelling kit (Cadema)
   (b) one 5 ml syringe
   (c) two 2 ml syringes
   (d) two green needles (21G)
   (e) white (1½ inch × 19G) special needle
   (f) one 2 ml ampoule of Disodium Edetate Inj. 4.4%
   (g) one 10 ml sterile, pyrogen-free vial
   (h) one lead pot
   (i) $^{99}Tc^m$-pertechnetate with activity of 370–740 MBq/ml
   Do *not* use the first elution from a new generator.
2. Using a 10 ml heparinized syringe with a (21G) green needle, draw 4 ml of blood from the patient with a clean venepuncture. Swab the rubber closure of the Red cell labelling kit with a chlorhexidine swab. Allow the partial vacuum in the tube to draw the blood into the kit.
3. Mix immediately to dissolve the solids by gently rotating the tube for 5 min.
4. Transfer 1 ml of Disodium Edetate Inj. 4.4% using the 2 ml syringe to the tube, first aspirating air to produce a vacuum, which will draw the solution into the tube. Repeat the aspiration if necessary.
5. Mix the contents of the tube by careful inversion several times.
6. Centrifuge the tube, *stopper down*, for 5 min at 1300*g* in the centrifuge. Remember the *balance* tube!
7. While the tube is centrifuging, transfer 1–3 ml of the pertechnetate containing 900–1100 MBq into the 10 ml vial using a 2 ml syringe and 21G needle.
8. After centrifuging, transfer the tube to the laminar flow cabinet, keeping the *stopper down* and *without shaking* to avoid disturbing the packed red blood cells. Swab the rubber closure thoroughly with chlorhexidine.
9. Using a 2 ml syringe and the special (1½ inch × 19G) white needle transfer 1.25 ml of the packed red blood cells from the tube into the vial containing the pertechnetate. This transfer must be done carefully so as not to disturb the layer of red blood cells in the tube. Insert the tip of the needle through the rubber stopper, and draw the cells into the syringe in one smooth continuous movement. Do not allow air to be drawn

into the tube, which will resuspend the cells. If this happens, repeat the centrifugation step.

10. Carefully invert the vial several times to mix and incubate the labelled red-blood-cell mixture for 5 min at room temperature.

11. Assay and label the vial with activity, volume, time, date, batch number and patient's name, and prepare two further identical labels, one for the record book and one for the patient's request form.

12. Complete a sheet in the blood products records book, including the following:
    (a) date
    (b) name of preparation
    (c) kit lot number
    (d) $^{99}Tc^m$ generator number
    (e) Disodium Edetate Inj. 4.4% lot number
    (f) total activity in the vial
    (g) volume
    (h) time
    (i) batch number

13. Attach a specimen label to the record sheet.

7.1.4 STANNOUS AGENT (FOR IN VIVO Tc-RBC LABELLING)

> **Note**
> *Aseptic procedure* Switch on the laminar flow cabinet at least 30 min before starting. Swab with 0.5% chlorhexidine in 70% spirit.

1. Collect the following:
   (a) vial of stannous agent
   (b) one 10 ml syringe
   (c) one 10 ml ampoule of 0.9% w/v sodium chloride for injections
   (d) swab (isopropyl alcohol or chlorhexidine)

2. Remove the central metal disc from the stannous agent vial.

3. Swab the rubber closures of the stannous agent vial and the neck of the glass ampoule.

4. Transfer the recommended volume of the saline into the stannous agent vial and withdraw an equal volume of gas from the vial.

5. Shake the vial for 1 min.

6. Label the vial with volume, time, date, batch number and expiry time.

7. The first patient dose may be removed from the vial up to 6 h after reconstitution. Subsequent patient doses must be removed *within* 2 h of removal of the first dose.

8. Record the following in the radiopharmaceuticals record book:
   (a) date
   (b) name of preparation

(c) stannous agent kit lot number
(d) volume
(e) time
(f) batch number

Warning
The. vial should *not* be reconstituted with pertechnetate from a technetium generator.

7.1.5 $^{99}Tc^m$-LABELLED HSA MICROSPHERES

Note
Aseptic procedure   Switch on the laminar flow cabinet at least 30 min before starting.

---

1. Collect the following:
   (a) vial of microspheres kit
   (b) lead pot
   (c) 10 ml syringe
   (d) pertechnetate
   (e) one 10 ml ampoule of 0.9 w/v sodium chloride for injections
   (f) swab (isopropyl alcohol or chlorhexidine)
   (g) ultrasonic bath containing ¾ inch of distilled water
2. Remove the central metal disc from the HSA microspheres labelling vial.
3. Swab the rubber closures of the labelling, pertechnetate and saline vials.
4. Place the labelling vial in the lead pot.
5. Transfer the manufacturer's recommended volume and activity of pertechnetate to the microspheres labelling vial.
6. Shake the vial vigoriously for 10 s.
7. Transfer the labelling vial from the lead pot to the ultrasonic bath.
8. Ultrasound for 5 min.
9. Assay and label the vial with activity, volume, time, date, batch number and expiry time.
10. Store at 2–8°C in the refrigerator and use within 6 h of preparation.
11. Record the following in the radiopharmaceuticals records book:
    (a) date of preparation
    (b) name of preparation
    (c) manufacturer's lot number
    (d) $^{99}Tc^m$ generator number
    (e) total activity in vial
    (f) volume
    (g) time
    (h) batch number

7.2 STRESS TESTING

> **Note**
> Stress testing must be carried out by or under the direct supervision of a medically qualified doctor.

The following equipment must be available if the test is to be carried out safely and efficiently:
1. ECG recording machine with a continuous ECG monitor.
2. Full resuscitation facilities, including a DC defibrillator.
3. Continuous blood pressure recordings using a cuff sphygmomanometer are used as an index of the ventricular response to stress.
4. A bicycle ergometer.

7.2.1 BICYCLE ERGOMETER EXERCISE PROCEDURE

Table 7.1   A ^{201}Tl cardiac stress/exercise worksheet.

Date of study	
Name	Consultant
Address	Hospital no.
	Date of birth
	Telephone

Clinical data and risk factors for CAD
Weight
Height
Tobacco
Lipids
Daily exercise

Family history of
CAD

Diabetes

Hypertension

History and medication

1. The clinical history, examination and resting ECG findings are always reviewed before starting the test, so that any necessary precautions can be taken and a limited study performed if clinically appropriate (Record these details on a cardiac stress worksheet (Table 7.1)).
2. An IV cannula is inserted in an antecubital arm vein, in the arm opposite to the one to be used for BP measurement and checked by flushing with heparinized saline to ensure patency.

Table 7.2   Bicycle ergometer exercise worksheet.

Name

Hospital and unit number
Consultant

Reason for referral
(a) Suspected CAD   ☐   (b) ?Significance of stenosis   ☐
(c) Assessment post-CABG   ☐   (d) Associated arrhythmia   ☐
(e) Other (specify)   ☐

Resting ECG
Rhythm   Rate   /min
                                    Axis

Comments

		Exercise test		
	BP	Pulse	Time	ECG changes
Rest				
25 W				
50 W				
75 W				
100 W				
125 W				
150 W				
175 W				
200 W				

Exercise stopped by   Total work performed   W min
   Chest pain ☐   Dyspnoea ☐
   Fatigue   ☐   Other   ☐   (specify)

Comments

3. ECG electrodes are attached to the patient's chest and a resting ECG recorded. The patient's baseline blood pressure and pulse are recorded (Table 7.2).
4. The bicycle seat is adjusted for patient comfort and the patient is instructed to cycle with the initial workload set at 25 W. Thereafter, the workload is increased every 2 min by 25 W until a standard endpoint has been achieved, i.e. patient forced to stop because of general fatigue, dyspnoea, chest pain, muscle fatigue or other symptoms.

   The ECG, pulse and BP measurements should be recorded every 2 min (Table 7.2).
5. The measured dose of ^{201}Tl is injected through the butterfly as soon as the endpoint is reached, and the patient is instructed to continue pedalling for a further 2 min at 25–50 W.
6. Final ECG, pulse and BP measurements are recorded at 2 min after the end of this procedure.

7.2.2 PERSANTIN STRESS PROCEDURE

Persantin (dipyridamole) stress is used for patients who are unsuitable for dynamic exercise. It should be used automatically for patients whose physical condition makes it obvious that they cannot exercise, and may be used at the doctor's discretion for patients who give up early having started exercise.

1. The patient is weighed.
2. ECG electrodes are attached and an ECG recorded.
3. An IV cannula (butterfly, venflon with tubing) is inserted and filled with saline.
4. A blood pressure cuff is attached to the patient's arm that does not have the IV cannula.
5. BP, pulse and ECG strips are recorded every minute throughout the procedure until hand grip is completed.
6. Trinitrin (glyceryl trinitrate) tablets (0.5 mg) and aminophylline (250 mg in 10 ml) must be available and ready for use.
7. With the patient sitting at rest, Persantin in a dose of 0.5 mg/kg is injected intravenously over 4 min. This is *critical* and the infusion must not be speeded up.
8. At the end of the 4 min infusion, the patient is exercised gently by walking on the spot for 6 min.
9. At the end of the 6 min exercise, the patient carries out isometric hand grip to 50% of maximum for 2 min.
10. Immediately following this the ^{201}Tl dose is injected IV and the cannula flushed, and handgrip is maintained for a further 1 min.
11. If at any stage the patient develops severe chest pain or potentially

dangerous cardiac dysrhythmia, the patient is given sublingual trinitrin. If the pain is not relieved rapidly, or the rhythm remains alarming, IV aminophylline is infused slowly until relief or maximum dose of 500 mg over 20 min has been given. If it is necessary to give trinitrin or aminophylline, the ^{201}Tl is given as soon as possible and the test ended at this point.

7.3 ^{201}Tl MYOCARDIAL IMAGING

7.3.1 PATIENT PREPARATION

The patients should be warned when the appointment is made that they will be carrying out an exercise test, and should be dressed accordingly. They should also be warned about the need to attend for delayed images.

If the patient has an obvious reason for not being able to exercise (e.g. one leg) or is unlikely to exercise adequately, then a dipyridamole stress should be used.

7.3.2 RADIOPHARMACEUTICAL AND DOSE

70 MBq ^{201}Tl-thallous chloride

The dose is injected intravenously at peak of exercise.

7.3.3 EQUIPMENT

A standard-field-of-view gamma camera is used, fitted with a general all-purpose (GAP) collimator. If a wide-field-of-view gamma camera is to be used, then the magnification mode should be selected.

A lead cape is used for masking out extracardiac activity and hence improve the image quality. It can be home-made from lead rubber (with 1 mm lead equivalent) by cutting out a 15 cm diameter circle from the centre of a piece measuring 30 cm square.

7.3.4 PATIENT POSITIONING

The patient is positioned supine on the imaging table for the anterior and left anterior oblique (LAO 45° and LAO 55°) views and on the right side with a pillow under the right side of the chest for the left lateral view, with the arms raised to ensure that the left arm is well clear of the chest.

7.3.5 COMPUTER

The computer is set up to record four static frames in a 128 × 128 word matrix for 10 min each, stopping on overflow. The desired amount of magnification should be selected before commencing acquisition on the computer.

7.3.6 TECHNIQUE

1. The patient is exercised using the standard exercise protocol (see Sections 7.2.1 and 7.2.2) and imaged as soon as possible after exercise.
2. Ensure camera, film back and computer are set. Select 30% window, centred on low-energy (85 keV) thallium peak.

3. Position patient as in patient positioning and record the anterior, left anterior obliques (LAO 45° and LAO 55°) and left lateral views for 10 min per view. The lead cape should be positioned carefully to ensure that no part of the myocardium is excluded. The position of the lead cape can be marked on the patient's chest to facilitate repositioning for delayed images.
4. The imaging procedure is repeated at 3–4 h. The number of views to be recorded may be selected by the physician on duty.

7.3.7 IMAGE LAYOUT

Anterior	LAO 45°
LAO 55°	Left lateral

The delayed set of images are recorded on a separate film using a similar layout.

Note
Currently there is a preference to record LAO 70° view instead of the LAO 55° and left lateral views.

7.3.8 ANALYSIS

Each image is background-subtracted using weighted bilinear interpolative background correction. The left ventricle is outlined, the geometric centre determined and area divided into $36 \times 10°$ segments. The same region is superimposed on the delayed image after correcting for change in position.

The counts in each segment are displayed as two pairs of circumferential profiles:
1. Exercise and delayed counts each normalized to their respective segment maxima to demonstrate changes in relative ²⁰¹TI distribution.
2. Exercise and delayed absolute counts in each segment.

The unprocessed images and the background-subtracted images are displayed together for exercise and delayed studies for each view in order to make a visual assessment of changes.

7.4 INFARCT IMAGING

7.4.1 PATIENT PREPARATION

There is no patient preparation.

7.4.2 RADIOPHARMACEUTICAL AND DOSE

350 MBq ^{99}Tc^m-pyrophosphate injected IV

7.4.3 EQUIPMENT

A standard-field-of-view gamma camera is used, fitted with a high-resolution collimator. A wide-field-of-view gamma camera may also be used, but should be set to magnify the image.

7.4.4 PATIENT POSITIONING

The patient is positioned supine on the imaging table for the anterior and left anterior oblique (LAO 45°) views and on the right side with a pillow under the right side of the chest for the left lateral view, with the arms raised to ensure that the left arm is well clear of the chest.

7.4.5 COMPUTER

The computer is set up to record each static view in a 128 × 128 word matrix, for 5 min per view.

7.4.6 TECHNIQUE

1. The patient is injected intravenously with the measured dose of ^{99}Tc^m-pyrophosphate.
2. Initial images are recorded at 2 h after injection. The patient is positioned for the anterior view as in patient positioning so that the sternum is half-way down the field of view and somewhat off-centre in order that the entire left side of the chest is included. This anterior view is recorded as a 5 min analogue image on film as well as the computer.
3. The LAO 45° and the left lateral images are also recorded for 5 min each, following the image layout below and the patient positioning as described earlier.
4. Delayed images are recorded at about 6 h after the initial injection, using

the same settings on the camera as those used for recording the 2 h images.

7.4.7 IMAGE LAYOUT

Anterior 2 h	Anterior 6 h
LAO 45° 2 h	LAO 45° 6 h
Left lateral 2 h	Left lateral 6 h

7.5 GATED RED-CELL STUDIES

7.5.1 PATIENT PREPARATION

There is no preparation required for adult patients. The very young patient will need to be adequately sedated if the study is to be carried out safely and efficiently.

7.5.2 RADIOPHARMACEUTICAL AND DOSE

750 MBq ^{99}Tc^m-RBCs

The adult dose is 750 MBq ^{99}Tc^m-labelled autologous red blood cells in a volume of 1–2 ml, and this is adjusted in children on the basis of body surface area.

If the facility for labelling red cells *in vitro* is not available, then the *in vivo* labelling method using stannous agent can be used:
1. Inject 0.03 ml/kg body weight of stannous agent.
2. Wait 30 min.
3. Inject the measured dose of ^{99}Tc^m-pertechnetate (adult dose = 750 MBq, adjusted in children on the basis of body surface area).
4. Wait 20 min before commencing equilibrium blood pool imaging.

7.5.3 PATIENT POSITIONING

The patient is positioned supine on the imaging table, with the camera centred over the chest (Fig. 7.1).

Accurate positioning can be achieved by using a ^{57}Co marker source attached to the suprasternal notch and positioning so that the marker appears dead centre at the top of the field of view.

7.5.4 EQUIPMENT

The study is ideally performed using a standard-field-of-view gamma camera (preferably a mobile gamma camera), fitted with a general all-purpose or high-resolution collimator. If a wide-field-of-view camera is to be used, then the camera should be set on 'Mag' and/or software zoom selected on the data system.

The LAO 45° views are best performed using a rotating slant-hole collimator, as this can be positioned to achieve good atrioventricular separation (Fig. 7.2).

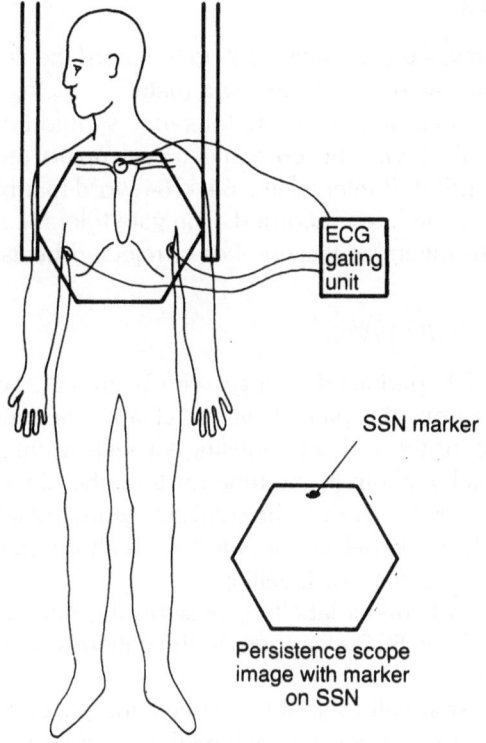

Fig. 7.1   Patient positioning for a gated red-cell study.

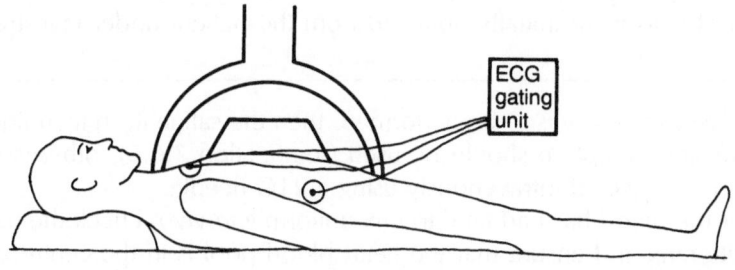

Fig. 7.2   Patient positioning for a LAO 45° gated red-cell study.

7.5.5 COMPUTER

For the anterior view, the computer is set up to record the desired numnber of frames per R–R interval in a 64 × 64 word matrix, stopping when 4 000 000 counts have been recorded. The gate tolerance should be set at 100 ms.

For the LAO 45° views, the computer is set up to record the desired number of frames per R–R interval in a 64 × 64 word matrix, stopping when 3 500 000 counts have been recorded. The gate tolerance should be set at 200 ms in order to minimize the number of rejected beats.

7.5.6 TECHNIQUE (*IN VIVO*)

1. Using a 10 ml heparinized syringe with a green (21G) needle, draw 4 ml of blood from the patient with a clean venepuncture. Swab the rubber closure of the red-cell labelling kit with a chlorhexidine swab. Allow the partial vacuum in the tube to draw the blood into the kit.

   Mix immediately to dissolve the solids by gently rotating the tube for 5 min. Do *not* shake. Label the sample tube with the patient's name and send it to the laboratory for labelling.
2. Whilst the blood is being labelled, position the patient on the imaging table, and attach the ECG electrodes to the patient's chest and connect to the gating unit.

   The gating signal will be much clearer if the patient's skin is cleaned with an alcohol swab prior to attaching the electrodes. Also keeping the ECG leads well clear of any mains leads will reduce mains interference.
3. Position patient for the anterior view as described earlier. Check the camera settings and set up the computer to acquire using the parameters listed above.

> **Note**
> Before injecting the red cells, ensure by checking against the label that the red cells were initially obtained from the patient under investigation.

4. If a first-pass study is to be performed, then the saline flush technique of bolus administration should be used (see Section 7.6.6), otherwise the patient is injected intravenously using a 21G needle.
5. After the blood has had time to mix uniformly *in vivo*, check the patient positioning and ensure that the heart blood pool is in the centre of the field of view, paying particular attention to the apex of the left ventricle, and record the equilibrium gated study.
6. Obtain a trace of the patient's ECG and check with a doctor on duty whether the patient can be stressed. If the patient is not a suitable

candidate for stressing (using supine exercise, hand grip or cold pressor), then record the left anterior oblique, right anterior oblique and left posterior oblique views using the same acquisition parameters as the anterior.

7.5.7 PROCEDURE FOR STRESS GATED CARDIAC

Note
The patient should not be stressed unless a doctor is supervising the stress study.

1. If the patient can be stressed, then attach a slant-hole (general all-purpose) collimator to the camera and angle the camera at 40°. Rotate the slant-hole collimator so that the plane of the slant hole is at 10° caudally. Position the camera against the patient's left side of chest and, using the persistence display on the computer, centre the image.

Table 7.3   A cardiac stress worksheet.

Date of study						
Name			Consultant			
Address			Hospital no.			
			Date of birth			
			Telephone			

Clinical data						
Weight			Drugs			
Height						
Tobacco						

Family history of			Present symptoms			
CAD						
Diabetes						
Hypertension						

	Cold pressor		Hand grip		Supine exercise	
	Pulse	BP	Pulse	BP	Pulse	BP
Rest						
1 min						
2 min						
3 min						
4 min						
5 min						

2. Adjust the gain (software or hardware) on the computer system so that only the left ventricle and as much of the right side of the heart blood pool including the right ventricle is in the field of view. It may be necessary to adjust the camera angle and for the collimator slant holes to be rotated to obtain good septal separation and to display an 'oval'-shaped left ventricular cavity. Once this is achieved, instruct the patient to remain still for the remainder of the study.
3. Set up the computer to record the cold pressor study using identical parameters to the resting LAO.
4. Record the patient's baseline BP and pulse on the cardiac worksheet (Table 7.3). If these are acceptable, then place the patient's left hand in the container full of ice and water.

   Start the computer acquisition at 45 s after the hand is placed in the ice. Run off a short trace of the patient's ECG. Record the patient's BP and pulse at 1 min intervals for the duration of the acquisition (Table 7.3).
5. If at any stage the patient develops chest pain or becomes short of breath, the procedure should be terminated.
6. When the acquisition is complete, remove the patient's hand from the ice and monitor the BP and pulse until they return to baseline values. Normally this takes about 5 min.

Isometric hand grip

Before proceeding to the next step, check using persistence that the patient has not moved significantly. If the patient has moved, then reposition the patient.

Set up the computer to record using identical parameters to the cold pressor and LAO resting studies.

When the patient's BP and pulse have returned to baseline values, establish the individual's workload level using the hand grip apparatus as follows:

1. Instruct the patient to grip the rubber ball of the hand grip apparatus (vigorometer) and to squeeze the rubber ball as hard as possible and then release it. This will determine the maximum pressure. Set the indicator level on the vigorometer to half this maximum value.
2. Tell the patient to squeeze the rubber ball with a firm grip of the hand and to maintain the pressure to the level already determined.
3. Start acquisition on the computer at 60–90 s after start of hand grip and run off a strip of the patient's ECG trace.
4. Throughout the study check that the patient maintains the predetermined pressure as, after the first 2 min, it becomes quite difficult. Record the patient's BP and pulse at 1 min intervals throughout the study (Table 7.3).

5. When the acquisition is complete, the patient should be rested until the BP and pulse have returned to baseline values. This usually takes about 5 min.

7.5.8 ANALYSIS

The most frequently measured parameter from a gated cardiac study is the left ventricular ejection fraction. This is calculated by a program that automatically or semi-automatically draws a region of interest around the left ventricle at end diastole and end systole and a background region. The ejection fraction is calculated as follows:

$$\text{LVEF (\%)} = \frac{\text{ED counts} - \text{ES counts}}{\text{ED counts} - \text{Background}} \times 100$$

where ED = end diastolic and ES = end systolic. This parameter can also be calculated on a regional basis by dividing the left ventricle into segments. These results assume that ventricular counts are proportional to ventricular volume. The change in wall motion can also be assessed quantitatively on a regional basis, and visually by looking at a ciné playback of the study.

Functional images can be calculated showing a number of functional parameters displayed pixel by pixel as a function of intensity. These parameters include stroke volume, ejection fraction, amplitude and phase.

Other phase measurements that can be made include peak ejection and filling rates measured from the left ventricular count–time curve, the ratio of left to right ventricular stroke volumes, which is useful for evaluating regurgitant valve disease, and right ventricular ejection fraction. The latter is probably most accurately calculated from a first-pass study, which provides temporal separation of the right ventricle from the left but is, even so, less reliable than the left ventricular ejection fraction.

7.6 FIRST-PASS STUDY FOR LEFT-TO-RIGHT SHUNT DETECTION

7.6.1 PATIENT PREPARATION

The majority of patients requiring this investigation are young children and infants, and will therefore need to be adequately sedated if the procedure is to be carried out safely and efficiently. The patient should be cannulated with a heparinized saline-filled syringe attached to the cannula to prevent the formation of clots.

7.6.2 RADIOPHARMACEUTICAL AND DOSE

750 MBq $^{99}Tc^m$-DTPA or $^{99}Tc^m$-RBCs

If the study is being performed to detect a shunt, then $^{99}Tc^m$-DTPA should be used. The adult dose is 750 MBq and should be corrected in children on the basis of their body surface area.

If a gated study is to be combined with the shunt study, then $^{99}Tc^m$-labelled autologous red blood cells should be used or the *in vivo* method of labelling red cells may be used. The doses are similar to the $^{99}Tc^m$-DTPA doses used for the shunt study.

7.6.3 EQUIPMENT

A standard-field-of-view gamma camera fitted with a general all-purpose collimator is used. For very young children, where the dose injected is very small in terms of activity, a high-sensitivity collimator should be used.

7.6.4 PATIENT POSITIONING

The patient is positioned supine on the imaging table with the camera centred over the heart. Accurate positioning should be obtained by using carefully positioned ^{57}Co marker sources.

If necessary, the patient should be immobilized using suitable restraining devices. Usually this is not necessary but the patients should be watched very carefully in case they should wake up or perform sudden movements and consequently cause injury whilst under the camera.

7.6.5 COMPUTER

The computer is set up to record information in gated list mode for 20 s. If the facility for list mode is not available, then record at two frames per second using a 64 × 64 byte matrix.

On some data systems the data are recorded at 32 frames per second instead of list mode. These data can then be regrouped to produce frames of any time interval desired, as with the list mode acquisition.

7.6.6 TECHNIQUE

> **Note**
>
> If only the nuclear angiogram (using $^{99}Tc^m$-DTPA) is to be performed, then proceed to step 3.

1. Using a 10 ml heparinized syringe with a green (21G) needle, draw 4 ml of blood from the patient with a clean venepuncture. Swab the rubber closure of the red-cell labelling kit with a chlorhexidine swab and allow the partial vacuum in the tube to draw the blood into the kit.

   Mix immediately to dissolve the solids by gently rotating the tube for 5 min. Do *not* shake. Label the sample tube with the patient's name and send it to the laboratory for labelling.

2. Whilst the blood is being labelled, position the patient on the imaging table, and attach the ECG electrodes to the patient's chest and connect to the gating unit.

   The gating signal will be much clearer if the patient's skin is cleaned with an alcohol swab prior to attaching the electrodes. Also keeping the ECG leads well clear of any mains leads will reduce mains interference.

3. The saline flush technique of bolus injection is used, as follows:

Injection technique

A special injection set is used for this technique. The set consists of an IV catheter, a three-way stopcock, a flexible connecting tube with luer lock fittings, a 20 ml syringe filled with 0.9% w/v sodium chloride solution for injections and a syringe containing the measured dose of the radio-pharmaceutical within a lead syringe shield.

Part of the injection set should be assembled prior to the vene-puncture. The flexible connecting tube is attached to the three-way stopcock and the syringe containing the saline flush attached to the opposite end of the stopcock. Air within the flexible tube and the stopcock is displaced with saline solution from the syringe. A tourniquet is applied around the patient's arm and the intravenous catheter is inserted into the antecubital vein.

When the venepuncture is successful, blood will flow back into the stylette. Release the tourniquet, remove the stylette from the catheter and connect the catheter to the flexible tubing. Flush through a small volume of the saline to ensure that the line is patent and to prevent possible formation of clots.

Position patient for the anterior view, check the camera settings and set up the computer to acquire using the parameters listed above.

Note
Before injecting the red cells check against the label to ensure that the red cells were initially obtained from the patient under investigation.

Attach the shielded syringe containing the labelled red cells to the three-way stopcock and introduce the dose through the stopcock into the extension tube. If the volume of the red cells is too large to be accommodated into the extension tube, then the remainder should be left in the syringe to be injected after the bolus injection has been made.

Open the valve in the stop cock between the saline-filled syringe and the extension tube and give a rapid injection of the saline to propel the dose into the vein. The injection should be rapid and steady so that an intact and compact bolus may be delivered.

4. Start the acquisition on the computer immediately before the bolus is injected.
5. If an equilibrium gated blood pool study is to be performed, then attach the general all-purpose collimator. Centre the camera over the patient's chest so that the heart blood pool is in the centre of the field of view. Adjust the zoom or gain on the computer and record 18 frames per R–R interval, for 3 500 000 conts.
6. Similarly record the LAO 45° using a slant-hole collimator, if available. Angle the detector so that it is angled along the septum with a 15° caudal tilt, giving the best delineation of the ventricles.

If the patient has congenital heart disease, the positioning may need to be modified.

7.6.7 ANALYSIS

The aim of the analysis is to calculate the size of the left-to-right shunt, usually expressed as the Q_p/Q_s ratio.

The first-pass study data are restructured into a dynamic study of two or four frames per second. This restructured study is analysed by drawing regions of interest over the superior vena cava (SVC) and the right lung field. The latter region is defined by subtracting a frame that shows the left ventricular phase well from a frame that shows the lungs clearly, leaving an image of the lungs only. Time–activity curves are generated for each region. The SVC curve should be inspected to determine if the bolus is good and, if it is not, the lung curve can be deconvoluted using the SVC curve as an input function.

By applying a least-squares fit of a gamma variate function of the lung curve, one can accurately estimate the pulmonary flow. The fitted curve is then subtracted from the raw data to give a pulmonary recirculation curve. A gamma variate is also fitted to this curve and the ratio of the area under the first transit curve to the area under the recirculation curve is the pulmonary/ systemic flow ratio (Q_p/Q_s).

Difficulty in shunt quantification is caused by the following factors:

1. Poor bolus injection.
2. SVC obstruction.
3. A large heart in a small chest, causing difficulty in placing a region of interest over the lung alone.
4. A single ventricle or a large VSD chamber mixing.

7.7 BLOOD FLOW STUDY FOR RIGHT-TO-LEFT SHUNT DETECTION

7.7.1 PATIENT PREPARATION

As with the left-to-right cardiac shunt study, the majority of patients requiring this investigation are young children and infants, and will therefore need to be adequately sedated if the procedure is to be carried out safely and efficiently.

The patient, unfortunately, cannot be cannulated prior to the injection of the $^{99}Tc^m$-microspheres since the microspheres tend to stick to plastic tubing.

7.7.2 RADIOPHARMACEUTICAL AND DOSE

$^{99}Tc^m$-microspheres

The injected dose should not contain more than 50 000 microspheres for a child. The radioactivity injected will depend on the concentration of the initial preparation. As a guide, the child's dose can be calculated assuming a standard adult dose of 100 000 microspheres:

$$\text{Child's dose} = \begin{array}{c}\text{Volume containing}\\ \text{100 000 microspheres}\end{array} \times \frac{\text{Child's surface area}}{1.73 \times 2}$$

> **Note**
> The dose of microspheres must not be drawn up in the syringe for any length of time prior to injecting since the microspheres tend to adhere to the wall of the syringe.

7.7.3 EQUIPMENT

A wide-field-of-view gamma camera fitted with a general all-purpose or high-resolution collimator is used.

7.7.4 PATIENT POSITIONING

The patient is positioned supine on the imaging table for the anterior views and prone for the posterior views. The camera is only placed under the imaging table if the patient is unable to lie prone.

If necessary, the patient should be immobilized using suitable restraining devices. Usually this is not necessary but the patients should be watched very carefully in case they wake up or perform sudden movements and consequently cause injury whilst under the camera.

7.7.5 COMPUTER

The computer is set up to record each static image in a 128 × 128 word matrix for 5 min per view.

7.7.6 TECHNIQUE

1. Shake the vial containing the ^{99}Tc^m-microspheres immediately before drawing up the calculated volume as indicated above.
2. Inject the dose with the patient positioned supine on the imaging table.
3. Commence imaging as soon as the dose has been injected, since rapid loss of ^{99}Tc^m occurs from the particles, possibly due to fragmentation, and a consequent overestimate of shunt size will occur.
4. Record images to cover the whole body, excluding the limbs, for 5 min per view. Both the lungs should be included in the anterior and posterior thorax views. If the field of view of the camera is not large enough to accommodate both lungs, then overlapping views should be recorded.

7.7.7 ANALYSIS

The aim of the analysis is to calculate the size of the right-to-left shunt.

Normally, the microspheres embolize in the pulmonary circulation and do not appear in the systemic circulation following an intravenous injection. If there is a right-to-left shunt, the microspheres appear in the systemic circulation.

Using irregular regions of interest, the counts from the lungs and the rest of the body can be obtained, and by substituting the values in the following, the shunt can be measured:

$$\text{Right-to-left shunt (\%)} = \frac{\text{TBC}-\text{TLC}}{\text{TBC}} \times 100$$

where TBC = total body counts and TLC = total lung counts.

CHAPTER EIGHT

NEUROLOGICAL STUDIES

INTRODUCTION

By routinely performing a cerebral flow study on patients having radio-nuclide brain scans, the number of differential diagnostic possibilities for a positive brain scan can be decreased as information on the vascularity of the lesion is available. Areas of grossly decreased or slowed blood flow can be detected by this method. Further additional information can be obtained by recording images within a few minutes of injection. This allows the visualization of the equilibrium vascular pattern within the head before the radiopharmaceutical has time to concentrate in the extracellular space.

This procedure is very limited in its ability to resolve individual vessels, and without data processing, the information obtained is only semi-quantitative.

Many conditions alter the blood–brain barrier and permit the localization of a radiopharmaceutical. These include conditions such as strokes, primary and metastatic brain tumours, intracerebral abscesses and subdural haematomas. The much higher sensitivity and specificity provided by a CT scan has meant that radionuclide brain scans are now less frequently performed.

Radionuclide cisternography is performed in patients with symptoms of normal pressure hydrocephalus and for detection of CSF leaks. CSF is produced primarily from the choroid plexuses located in the lateral, third and fourth ventricles of the brain. ^{111}In-DTPA is used because of its longer half-life, since it is desirable to image the patient for 3–4 d.

8.1 RADIOPHARMACEUTICALS

8.1.1 $^{99}Tc^m$-GHA

> **Note**
> *Aseptic procedure*   Switch on the laminar flow cabinet at least 30 min before starting. Swab with 0.5% chlorhexidine in 70% spirit.

1. Collect the following:
   (a) one vial of GHA kit
   (b) one lead pot
   (c) one 10 ml syringe with 21G (green) needle
   (d) pertechnetate having the desired activity in 3–7 ml
   (e) one swab (isopropyl alcohol or chlorhexidine)
2. Remove the central metal disc from the GHA labelling vial.
3. Swab the rubber closures of the labelling and pertechnetate vials.
4. Place the labelling vial in the lead pot.
5. Transfer the manufacturer's recommended volume and activity of $^{99}Tc^m$-pertechnetate into the labelling vial. Withdraw an equal volume of gas from the vial.
6. Swirl the labelling vial for several seconds to dissolve completely.
7. Assay and label the vial with activity, volume, time, date, batch number and expiry time.
8. Use within the recommended shelf-life.
9. Record the following in the radiopharmaceutical records book
   (a) date
   (b) name of preparation
   (c) manufacturer's lot number
   (d) $^{99}Tc^m$-generator number
   (e) total activity in vial
   (f) volume
   (g) time
   (h) batch number

8.1.2 ^{111}In-DTPA

This is obtained ready for use as individual patient doses. Only an unopened ampoule should be used for cisternography. The only procedure necessary for dispensing is to check the activity in the ampoule against the label, and to check the expiry date.

8.1.3 $^{99}Tc^m$-PERTECHNETATE

This is obtained from the $^{99}Tc^m$ generator and it may be necessary to dilute it using 0.9% w/v sodium chloride for injections.

8.2 CEREBRAL FLOW STUDY

8.2.1 PATIENT PREPARATION

Nil.

8.2.2 RADIOPHARMACEUTICAL AND DOSE

750 MBq $^{99}Tc^m$-GHA, injected as IV bolus

The same activity of $^{99}Tc^m$-DTPA or $^{99}Tc^m$-pertechnetate may also be used. If $^{99}Tc^m$-pertechnetate is used, then the patient should be given 400 mg of potassium perchlorate, orally, immediately before or after the injection.

8.2.3 PATIENT POSITIONING

The patient is positioned supine on the imaging table.

For the anterior blood flow, the patient is positioned with the camera centred over the forehead to include as much of the neck as possible, with the radiologic baseline at right angles to the face of the collimator. For this reason the patient's head needs to be elevated by using two pillows under the head.

For the posterior view, the patient is positioned so that the patient lies with the back of the head on the camera face. Most of the patient's neck should be in the field of view of the camera. Again the radiologic baseline is used as a reference.

For the vertex view, the vertex 'lead cape' is used to shield the shoulders. The patient is positioned so that the head is just over the edge of the imaging table with the neck extended and the camera face parallel to the radiologic baseline.

In all cases care should be taken to ensure that the positioning is symmetrical.

8.2.4 EQUIPMENT

The study is performed on a standard-field-of-view camera fitted with a high-sensitivity collimator, or a wide-field-of-view camera may be used with a certain amount of zoom.

8.2.5 COMPUTER

The study is recorded on the computer at one frame per second for 40 s using a 64 × 64 byte matrix.

8.2.6 TECHNIQUE

1. Ensure camera, multiformatter and computer are set.
2. Position patient to image appropriate view as described under patient positioning.
3. Give bolus injection of $^{99}Tc^m$-GHA, starting computer at moment of cuff release.
4. At 2 min after injection, record the equilibrium image on camera for 300 000 counts.
5. The patient is then asked to return 90 min later for the static imaging part of the study.

8.2.7 IMAGE LAYOUT

Position 2 of the static brain imaging layout is used for recording the equilibrium image (see Section 8.3.7).

8.2.8 ANALYSIS

The flow study is analysed by drawing regular (or rectangular) regions of interest, of identical size, within the right and left cerebral hemispheres. Time–activity curves are generated of each region and a hard-copy image recorded (Fig. 8.1).

Three second vascular phase images are also recorded.

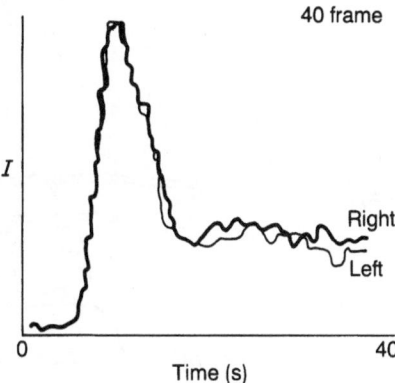

Fig. 8.1   Time–activity curves from a cerebral flow study.

8.3 STATIC BRAIN IMAGING

8.3.1 PATIENT PREPARATION

Nil.

8.3.2 RADIOPHARMACEUTICAL AND DOSE

750 MBq $^{99}Tc^m$-GHA, injected as IV bolus

The same activity of $^{99}Tc^m$-DTPA or $^{99}Tc^m$-pertechnetate may also be used. If $^{99}Tc^m$-pertechnetate is used, then the patient should be given 400 mg of potassium perchlorate, orally, immediately before or after the injection.

8.3.3 PATIENT POSITIONING

The patient is positioned supine for all views (Fig. 8.2). The positioning for all the views is the same as described in the cerebral flow study except that this time as little as possible of the face and neck should be in the field of view.

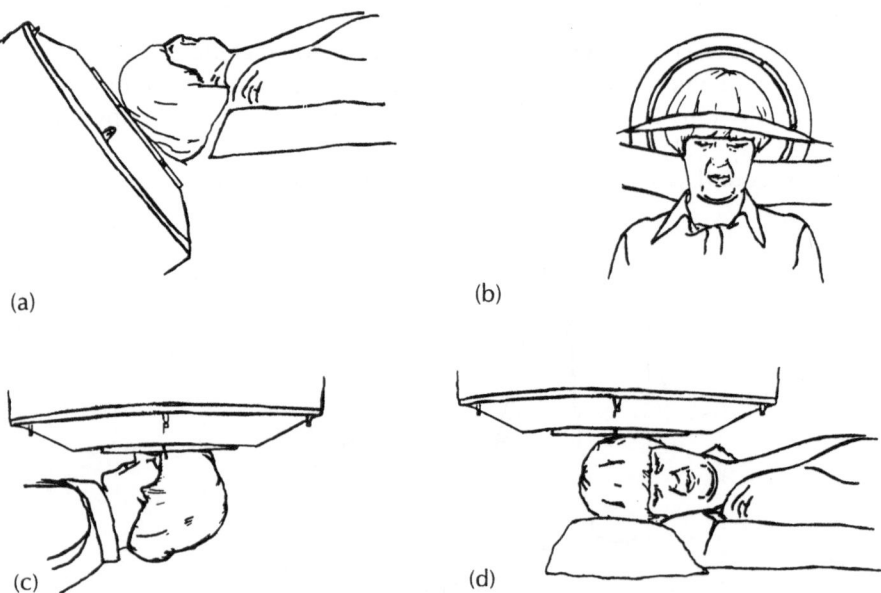

(a)

(b)

(c)

(d)

Fig. 8.2   Patient positioning for a static brain imaging study: (a) vertex; (b) posterior; (c) anterior; (d) lateral.

8.3.4 EQUIPMENT

A standard-field-of-view camera fitted with a GAP or a high-resolution collimator is ideal. If a wide-field-of-view camera is to be used, then a certain amount of zoom should be selected.

8.3.5 COMPUTER

The computer is not needed for this part of the study, but can be used for backing up the studies if the facility is available. The images should be recorded using a 128 × 128 word matrix for the same length of time or counts as the analogue images.

8.3.6 TECHNIQUE

1. The patient is positioned as described in patient positioning.
2. The anterior and posterior views are recorded for 300 000 counts each.
3. For the lateral views, the first lateral is recorded for 300 000 counts (this set count value should be increased depending on how much of the facial activity is in the field of view) and the time taken is noted. This preset time is then used for recording the other lateral.
4. For the vertex view, a 'lead cape' is used to mask out the activity from the shoulders and the image is recorded for 250 000 counts.

8.3.7 IMAGE LAYOUT

Anterior	Equilibrium
Right lateral	Left lateral
Posterior	Vertex

Note
In patients suspected of having subdurals, image at 3 h following injection as this gives a better target to non-target ratio.

8.4 CISTERNOGRAPHY

8.4.1 PATIENT PREPARATION

None, unless the study is being performed to detect cerebrospinal fluid (CSF) leaks, in which case nasal and pharyngeal packs must be positioned in place before injecting the radiopharmaceutical.

8.4.2 RADIOPHARMACEUTICAL AND DOSE

30 MBq ^{111}In-DTPA

An *unopened* ampoule must be used to ensure sterility of the ^{111}In-DTPA.

8.4.3 PATIENT POSITIONING

The patient is positioned supine for all the images. Following the injection, the patient is normally confined to bed for 24 h.

8.4.4 EQUIPMENT

A wide-field-of-view gamma camera is used, fitted with a medium-energy collimator.

8.4.5 COMPUTER

The studies are recorded on the computer for 7 min per view using a 128 × 128 word matrix. Images at later times should be recorded for 10 min per view.

8.4.6 TECHNIQUE

1. The radiopharmaceutical is introduced via a lumbar intrathecal injection. This is usually performed by the doctor on the ward, followed by bed rest for 24 h.
2. The site of injection should be imaged at the first visit to establish that the injection has been intrathecal. The patient is imaged at 2, 6, 24 and 48 h after injection. It may also be necessary to image at 72 h if indicated.
3. The anterior and one lateral view are always recorded, but if possible, both laterals, posterior and vertex views should be done. All images are

recorded for 7 min per view. Record the 72 h images for 10 min per view to compensate for the decay in ^{111}In.

8.4.7 IMAGE LAYOUT

Anterior	Posterior
Right lateral	Left lateral
Vertex	

Final image layout at the end of the study is obtained from the data system. The image layout for each view is as follows:

2 h	6 h
24 h	48 h
72 h	

8.4.8 ANALYSIS

Nil.

8.5 VENTRICULOATRIAL SHUNTS

8.5.1 PATIENT PREPARATION

The patient may need to be sedated.

8.5.2 RADIOPHARMACEUTICAL AND DOSE

37 MBq of ^{99}Tc^m-DTPA in 0.1 ml

8.5.3 PATIENT POSITIONING

The patient is positioned supine with the head turned to face the opposite side to that of the shunt, with the camera positioned above to include the shunt reservoir and the distal end of the tube.

8.5.4 EQUIPMENT

The study is performed on a wide-field-of-view gamma camera, fitted with a general all-purpose or high-resolution collimator.

8.5.5 COMPUTER

The computer is set up to record one frame per minute for 30 min using a 64 × 64 word matrix.

8.5.6 TECHNIQUE

1. Ensure camera, film back and computer are set.
2. The patient is positioned on the imaging table and the radiopharmaceutical injected into the shunt reservoir under sterile conditions.
3. As soon as the injection is complete, position the patient under the camera with the shunt side uppermost and lower the camera as close to the patient as possible to include the whole length of the shunt tube.
4. Start the computer acquisition and ensure that the patient remains still.
5. Record images every 5 min of 2 min duration each on film up to 30 min. Later images may need to be recorded if no activity is visible in the distal end of the tube at 30 min after injection.

8.5.7 IMAGE LAYOUT

0 min	5 min
10 min	15 min
20 min	25 min

8.5.8 ANALYSIS

The study is analysed by adding up all the images and defining a region of interest over the shunt reservoir. A time–activity curve of this region is then generated and recorded on hard copy for the report.

CHAPTER NINE

ENDOCRINE STUDIES

INTRODUCTION

In the early days of nuclear medicine, thyroid imaging and uptake used to constitute the main workload of most nuclear medicine departments. They are now well-established tests for evaluating many thyroid diseases, such as goitres, nodules, substernal masses and hyperthyroidism. $^{99}Tc^m$-pertechnetate can be used intravenously and the image obtained within 30 min following injection. The uptake of $^{99}Tc^m$ by the thyroid gland can be quantitated easily and provides additional valuable information.

^{123}I-Sodium iodide should be used for patients with retrosternal extensions since the iodine is avidly trapped and organified by the thyroid gland with no cardiac blood pool background as is seen with $^{99}Tc^m$-pertechnetate images.

Organification defects can be detected by performing a perchlorate discharge test. This involves administering a large oral dose (1 g) of potassium perchlorate to the patient after recording a baseline ^{123}I image and uptake. Any unorganified ^{123}I in the thyroid gland will be discharged following administration of the potassium perchlorate. Less than 10 % discharge is considered to be normal.

With all thyroid imaging studies, recent X-ray studies with contrast media and iodine-containing drugs the patient may have had, interfere with the uptake and this should be checked prior to the examination.

Well-differentiated thyroid cancers usually retain the ability to concentrate radioiodine. This allows the extent of the disease to be determined with a whole body radioiodine scan following total thyroidectomy. Prior to the follow-up scans, the patient is taken off oral thyroxine for four weeks, and the resultant hypothyroidism may make the patient feel unwell. Other alternative imaging agents, which can be used without the patient having to come off thyroxine, are being researched. Radioiodine contamination of the patient's skin and clothing can give rise to imaging artefacts and a check should always be made for this.

Parathyroid imaging is a recently introduced test used for the localization of functioning parathyroid adenomas in the neck and upper mediastinum. The test is usually performed in patients with definite biochemical evidence of hyperparathyroidism and is of great help to surgeons in planning operative procedure. Combined imaging with $^{99}Tc^m$-pertechnetate and ^{201}Tl is performed and since ^{201}Tl is taken up by the thyroid and parathyroid adenomata, computer subtraction of the $^{99}Tc^m$ image from the ^{201}Tl image will reveal the site of the adenoma.

Adrenal imaging is performed to diagnose adrenal hyperplasia, adenomas and carcinomas using ^{75}Se-methylcholesterol. For localizing phaeochromo-cytomas, ^{131}I-*meta*-iodobenzylguanidine (MIBG) is used.

The differential diagnosis of epididymitis and testicular torsion is clinically not always easy. The testicular scan allows a rapid, accurate and simple diagnosis to be made so that appropriate therapy can be rapidly instituted.

9.1 RADIOPHARMACEUTICALS

9.1.1 $^{99}Tc^m$-PERTECHNETATE

This is eluted from the $^{99}Tc^m$ generator and may require dilution with 0.9% w/v sodium chloride for injections to give approximately 350 MBq/ml. The dilution should be carried out in the laminar flow cabinet.

9.1.2 ^{123}I

> **Note**
> This procedure must be carried out in the designated fume cupboard.

Formula

^{123}I	20 MBq
Water for injection	10 ml

Materials

1. 20 MBq ^{123}I.
2. 10 ml water for injection.
3. 30 ml Sterilin vial.
4. Lead pot for iodine drinks.
5. 1 ml syringe with 21G needle.
6. 10 ml syringe with 21G needle.
7. Swab.
8. Drinks trolley.

Procedure

1. Swab the rubber closure of the ^{123}I vial and the neck of the glass ampoule of water for injection.
2. Using the 1 ml syringe withdraw sufficient water for injection and transfer to the ^{123}I vial to make a total volume of 1 ml in the vial.
3. Calculate the volume of diluted ^{123}I to give 20 MBq and transfer this volume using the same 1 ml syringe to the Sterilin vial contained in the lead pot.
4. Using the 10 ml syringe, transfer water for injection to the Sterilin vial to give a final volume of 10 ml.
5. Cap the Sterilin vial and check the radioactivity.
6. Label the Sterilin vial and the lid of the lead pot with:

(a) name of preparation
(b) date
(c) time
(d) total activity
(e) volume
(f) batch number (from ^{123}I vial)

7. Prepare the iodine drinks trolley with a clean sheet of Benchkote in the tray. Place the labelled lead pot containing the drink on the tray together with a straw, gloves and container of tap water.

8. After the drink has been administered, rinse the Sterilin vial twice with tapwater and carefully discard each of the washings into the designated sluice. Flush the sluice. Discard the Sterilin vial into the non-radioactive waste container. Rinse the syringe and needle in the sluice and discard.

9.1.3 ^{131}I

> **Note**
> This procedure must be carried out in the designated fume cupboard.

Formula

^{131}I (927 MBq/ml)	q.s.
Water for injection	10 ml

Materials

1. ^{131}I (quantity as requested on the form).
2. 10 ml water for injection.
3. 30 ml Sterilin vial.
4. Lead pot for iodine drinks.
5. One 1 ml syringe with (21G) green needle.
6. One 10 ml syringe with (21G) green needle.
7. One swab, isopropyl alcohol.
8. Drinks trolley.

Procedure

1. Swab the rubber closure of the ^{131}I vial and the neck of the glass ampoule of water for injection.
2. Calculate the volume of ^{131}I required. It will be necessary to select the appropriate ^{131}I vial using the record cards. Dilution of the ^{131}I with water for injection in the vial may be necessary to give a suitable volume.

3. Transfer the measured quantity of ^{131}I using the 1 ml syringe to the Sterilin vial contained in the lead pot.
4. Using the 10 ml syringe, transfer water for injection to the Sterilin vial to give a final volume of 10 ml.
5. Cap the Sterilin vial and check the radioactivity.
6. Label the Sterilin vial and the lid of the lead pot with:
   (a) name of preparation
   (b) date
   (c) time
   (d) total activity
   (e) volume
   (f) batch number (from ^{131}I vial)
7. Prepare the iodine drinks trolley with a clean sheet of Benchkote in the tray. Place the labelled lead pot containing the drink on the tray together with a straw, gloves and container of tap water.
8. After the drink has been administered, rinse the Sterilin vial twice with tap water and carefully discard each of the washings into the sluice to avoid splashing. Flush the sluice and discard the Sterilin vial into the non-radioactive waste container. Rinse the syringe and needle in the sluice and discard.

9.1.4 ^{75}Se-SELENOCHOLESTEROL (SCINTADREN)

This is obtained ready for use as individual patient doses. It is only necessary to check the activity in the vial against the label, and to check the expiry date.

9.1.5 ^{201}Tl-THALLOUS CHLORIDE

This is received ready for use, and the only procedure necessary is to measure and check the total activity in the vial against the label.

9.2 ^{99}Tc^m-THYROID IMAGING AND UPTAKE

9.2.1 PATIENT PREPARATION

Recent contrast X-ray studies and iodine-containing drugs, such as T4 and certain skin preparations, that the patient may have had interfere with uptake and this should be checked for.

9.2.2 RADIOPHARMACEUTICAL AND DOSE

180 MBq ^{99}Tc^m-Pertechnetate injected IV

9.2.3 EQUIPMENT

The study may be performed on a standard- or wide-field-of-view gamma camera fitted with a pinhole or a snout collimator. A Perspex neck phantom and foam block are also needed.

9.2.4 PATIENT POSITIONING

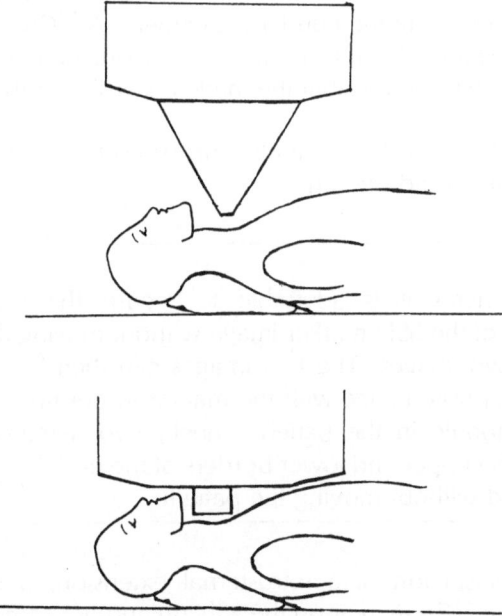

Fig. 9.1 Patient positioning for a thyroid imaging study: (a) using a pinhole collimator; (b) using a snout collimator.

The patient is positioned supine with a pillow under the shoulders so that the neck is well extended (Fig. 9.1).

9.2.5 COMPUTER

The syringe study is recorded for 1 min duration in a 64 × 64 word matrix, closing on overflow. The patient study is recorded for 100 000 counts or 15 min duration in a 64 × 64 word matrix.

9.2.6 TECHNIQUE

1. The patient doses are drawn up into numbered 1 ml syringes, a new needle attached and placed in the lead pot.
2. Each syringe in turn is placed in the phantom, the spacing adjusted with the foam block and the thyroid syringe recorded on the computer.
3. The patient is injected intravenously with the dose, and the syringe is flushed twice to ensure that all the measured activity is injected. The number of the syringe is written on the patient's request form.
4. The patient then waits for a minimum of 20 min.
5. Immediately prior to positioning the patient under the camera, the patient is given a drink of water to wash away activity from the oesophagus, and positioned under the camera. A ^{57}Co marker source is attached to the patient's suprasternal notch. Using persistence, the image is centred on the screen so that the marker is visible at the bottom of the field of view.
6. Record this image on the computer for 100 000 counts. An analogue image is also recorded on film.

Note

On digital cameras it is advisable to record the thyroid image independently of the SSN marker image without moving the patient in between the two images. The two images can then be added up to produce a composite image with the marker in position.

If there is a nodule in the patient's neck, two markers should be positioned at the upper and lower borders of the nodule, and a further image recorded without moving the patient.

---

7. If there is a suspicion of a retrosternal extension, a further view is recorded with a ^{57}Co marker on the SSN on another camera fitted with a general all-purpose or high-resolution collimator.
8. Oblique views are ideally performed using the pinhole collimator.

9.2.7 ANALYSIS

The study is analysed by carefully outlining the thyroid and defining a background area using irregular regions of interest excluding any other regions such as the salivary glands.

The background region should be chosen so that it lies within the patient's neck boundary and well away from the midline to avoid oesophageal activity.

By substituting the values in the following, the thyroid uptake can be calculated:

$$\text{Uptake (\%)} = \frac{TR - Bkgd}{SC \times DC} \times 100$$

where TR = thyroid region of interest counts per second, Bkgd = background counts per second with background region of interest normalized to thyroid region of interest, SC = counts per second of dose measured in syringe pre-injection using a thyroid phantom, and DC = decay correction factor obtained from table or graph for ^{99}Tc^m used to correct for the time lapse between measuring the pertechnetate and imaging the patient.

9.3 ^{123}I THYROID IMAGING AND UPTAKE

9.3.1 PATIENT PREPARATION

Recent contrast X-ray studies and iodine-containing drugs, such as T4 and certain skin preparations, that the patient may have had interfere with uptake and this should be checked for.

9.3.2 RADIOPHARMACEUTICAL AND DOSE

20 MBq ^{123}I-iodide administered as a drink

9.3.3 EQUIPMENT

The study may be performed on any camera fitted with a pinhole collimator or a snout collimator. The Perspex neck phantom and foam block are also needed. If the study is being done for a retrosternal extension, then a general all-purpose or high-resolution collimator is used.

9.3.4 PATIENT POSITIONING

The patient is positioned supine with a pillow under the shoulders so that the neck is well extended.

9.3.5 COMPUTER

The drink is recorded as a one frame static for 1 min in a 64 × 64 word matrix closing on overflow. The patient study is recorded for 200 000 counts or 15 min, whichever is the fastest. It is recorded in 64 × 64 word matrix, closing frame on overflow.

9.3.6 TECHNIQUE

1. The patient dose is placed in the neck phantom, the spacing adjusted with the foam block and the study is recorded on the computer.
2. The patient is given the dose using a straw, and the container rinsed with water to ensure that all the measured activity is drunk by the patient.
3. The patient then waits for a minimum of 2 h.
4. Before imaging, the patient is given a drink of water to wash away activity from the oesophagus, and positioned under the camera at the right distance using the foam spacer. A ^{57}Co marker source is attached to

the patient's suprasternal notch. Using persistence, the image is centred in the screen so that the marker is visible at the bottom of the field of view.

5. This image is recorded on the computer for 200 000 counts. An analogue image is also recorded on film.

Note

If there is a nodule in the patient's neck, two markers should be positioned at the upper and lower borders of the nodule, and a further image recorded without moving the patient.

On digital cameras it is advisable to record the thyroid image independently of the SSN marker image without moving the patient in between the two images. The two images can then be added up to produce a composite image with the marker in position.

---

6. If a retrosternal extension is suspected, a further view is recorded with a ^{57}Co marker on the SSN on another camera fitted with a general all-purpose collimator or high-resolution collimator.

9.3.7 ANALYSIS

The study is analysed by carefully outlining the thyroid and defining a background region using irregular regions of interest. By substituting the values in the following, the thyroid uptake can be calculated:

$$\text{Uptake (\%)} = \frac{\text{TR} - \text{Bkgd}}{\text{SC} \times \text{DC}} \times 100$$

where TR = thyroid region of interest counts per second, Bkgd = background counts per second with background region of interest normalized to thyroid region of interest, SC = counts per second of dose measured using a thyroid phantom, and DC = decay correction factor obtained from table or graph for the ^{123}I used to correct for the time lapse between measuring the drink and imaging the patient.

9.4 ^{123}I-PERCHLORATE DISCHARGE TEST

9.4.1 PATIENT PREPARATION

Recent contrast X-ray studies and iodine-containing drugs, such as T4 and certain skin preparations, that the patient may have had interfere with uptake and this should be checked for.

9.4.2 RADIOPHARMACEUTICAL AND DOSE

20 MBq ^{123}I
1 g potassium perchlorate (5 × 200 mg) dissolved in water

Orange squash may be added to make the preparation more palatable.

9.4.3 EQUIPMENT

The study may be performed on a standard- or a wide-field-of-view gamma camera fitted with a pinhole collimator.

9.4.4 PATIENT POSITIONING

The patient is positioned supine with a pillow under the shoulders so that the neck is well extended.

9.4.5 COMPUTER

The computer is set up to record 30 frames at one frame per minute in a 64 × 64 matrix, word mode.

9.4.6 TECHNIQUE

1. The patient is given the dose of ^{123}I using a straw, and the container rinsed with water to ensure that all the measured activity is drunk by the patient.
2. The patient is then asked to return 2 h later for imaging.
3. Before imaging, the patient is given a drink of water to wash away activity from the oesophagus, and positioned under the camera at the right distance using the foam spacer. A ^{57}Co marker source is attached to the patient's suprasternal notch. Using persistence, the image is centred in the screen so that the marker is at the bottom of the field of view.
4. The computer is set up and acquisition is started.

5. At 10 min, the patient is given the oral dose of potassium perchlorate to drink through a flexistraw, without moving.

9.4.7 ANALYSIS

The purpose of the analysis is to generate a time–activity curve of the thyroid region of interest to see whether the perchlorate discharges any free iodide present in the thyroid. This occurs if an organification defect is present.

The 30 frame dynamic study is summed up to produce a composite image and the thyroid is outlined using an irregular ROI. A time–activity curve of this region is plotted. A 10% drop in activity indicates a positive discharge.

9.5 ^{131}I WHOLE-BODY IMAGING

9.5.1 PATIENT PREPARATION

The patient is taken off oral T4 for 4 weeks or T3 for 2 weeks prior to the scan and put on a low-iodine diet. T4, thyroid-stimulating hormone (TSH) and thyroglobulin (TG) levels are measured before the patient attends for the drink.

9.5.2 RADIOPHARMACEUTICAL AND DOSE

^{131}I-sodium iodide

The dose is as prescribed by the physician. It is usually in the range of 37–555 MBq, depending on whether the patient is being treated or surveyed prior to treatment.

9.5.3 EQUIPMENT

A wide-field-of-view camera fitted with a medium-energy collimator is used. Images are backed up onto a data system if available.

9.5.4 PATIENT POSITIONING

The patient is positioned supine on the imaging table with the camera above, for the anterior views (Fig. 9.2).

For the posterior views, the patient lies prone (Fig. 9.2). If the patient is unable to lie prone, then the posterior views are recorded with the patient supine and the camera positioned below the imaging table.

9.5.5 COMPUTER

This is used if available and is set up to acquire static images in a 128 × 128 word matrix for 5 min per view.

9.5.6 TECHNIQUE

1. The patient is given the dose using a straw, and the container rinsed with water to ensure that all the measured activity is drunk by the patient.
2. The patient is then asked to return after 72 to 96 h depending on the camera schedule. The patient should be asked to have a shower and a

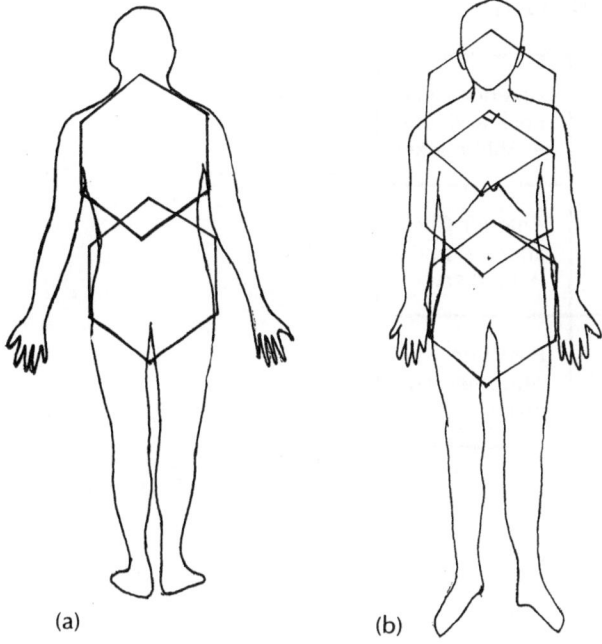

Fig. 9.2   Patient positioning for ^{131}I whole-body imaging: (a) posterior; (b) anterior.

fresh change of clothing on the morning of the scan in order to minimize the scan artifacts caused by iodine contamination of the skin and clothing.

3. Before commencing the scan, the patient should be asked to empty the bladder.
4. Static images of 5 min each are recorded to cover the whole body from nose to mid-femora, both anteriorly and posteriorly.
5. Two additional views with markers are always recorded:
   (a) to show the relative position of the SSN, by placing a ^{57}Co marker on the SSN and peaking the camera on ^{57}Co;
   (b) to show the position of the costal margins on the anterior abdomen view, by placing a ^{57}Co marker source on the patient's xiphisternum and two more on the right and left lower costal margins.

The marker images need only be recorded for 60 s duration each. These marker images can then be added to the corresponding images using the data system before recording the hard-copy images.

9.5.7 IMAGE LAYOUT

Anterior Head, neck and chest	Anterior Head, neck and chest + SSN marker
Anterior Chest and abdomen	Anterior Chest and abdomen + markers
Anterior Abdomen and pelvis	Posterior Abdomen and pelvis

9.6 PARATHYROID IMAGING

9.6.1 PATIENT PREPARATION

Nil.

9.6.2 RADIOPHARMACEUTICALS AND DOSES

70 MBq ^{201}Tl-thallous chloride
100 MBq ^{99}Tc^m-pertechnetate

The thallous chloride comes in a vial containing a nominal 250 MBq. Each vial contains enough for three patients and the actual dose should be checked in the dose calibrator after it is drawn up.

A butterfly set with a normal saline syringe is used for injecting.

9.6.3 EQUIPMENT

Any gamma camera fitted with a pinhole or a snout collimator may be used. Alternatively a small-field-of-view gamma camera fitted with a general all-purpose collimator may be used if a larger area is to be imaged, for example to include the mediastinum.

9.6.4 PATIENT POSITIONING

The patient is positioned supine with a pillow under the shoulder with the neck fully extended so that it is possible to have the camera as close as possible to the patient's neck (Fig. 9.3).

If a pinhole or a snout collimator is to be used, ^{57}Co marker sources are attached to the patient's suprasternal notch and chin. Using persistence, the patient is positioned so that the markers appear at the top and bottom of the image in the midline.

9.6.5 COMPUTER

If necessary, before positioning the patient, store uniformity correction images for the two radionuclides to be used. The computer is set up to record at one frame per minute for 15 min following each individual injection, using a 64 × 64 word matrix.

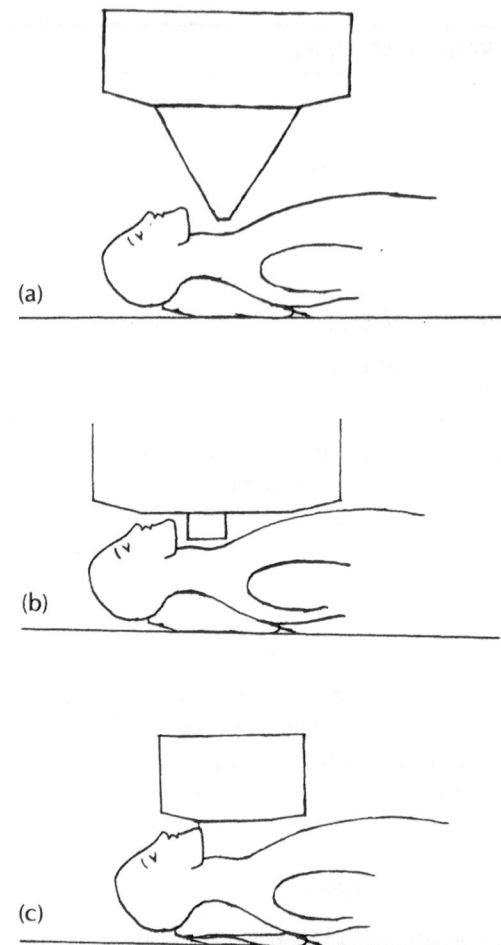

Fig. 9.3   Patient positioning for parathyroid imaging: (a) using a pinhole collimator; (b) using a snout collimator; (c) using a small-field-of-view gamma camera fitted with a GAP collimator.

9.6.6 TECHNIQUE (^{201}Tl INJECTION FIRST)

1. Ensure computer is set.
2. Position patient as described earlier and lock the trolley brakes. A head clamp may be used to prevent the patient from moving the head.
3. Store a marker view image for 30 s with the camera peaked on ^{57}Co, and mark the position of the markers on the persistence scope and the patient's skin for later reference. Remove the markers.

4. Set up the computer to record one frame per minute for 15 min. Peak the camera on ^{201}Tl (30% window).
5. Inject the patient intravenously with the measured dose of ^{201}Tl and wait 60 s before starting acquisition.
   If the positioning is incorrect then halt the acquisition, reposition and restart as soon as possible.
6. When acquisition is complete, peak the camera on ^{99}Tc^m, inject the patient intravenously with the measured dose of ^{99}Tc^m-pertechnetate and wait 60 s before starting acquisition. Record at one frame per minute for 15 min.
7. When acquisition is complete, reposition the markers and record an image for 30 s as before. If the patient has moved significantly since the start of the study, this image can be used for movement correction if necessary during analysis.
8. Throughout the study, make sure the patient keeps still, otherwise the subtraction is useless.

9.6.7 ANALYSIS (^{201}Tl FIRST)

1. Convert the 15 frame ^{201}Tl dynamic into a static frame. It may be necessary to ignore the first two frames.
2. Convert the technetium study into a static frame. Again, it may be necessary to ignore the first two frames. Also ignore the frames where the patient may have moved.
3. Outline the thyroid region using an irregular region of interest. Do this as accurately as possible and make a note of the total counts within this region (TC).
4. Select the summed-up thallium image and superimpose the technetium image region of interest on top of it. Note the total counts (TL).
5. Work out the correction factor for the ^{99}Tc^m image as follows:

$$^{99}\text{Tc}^m \text{ correction factor, CF} = \frac{\text{Total thallium ROI counts}}{\text{Total technetium ROI counts}} = \frac{\text{TL}}{\text{TC}}$$

This is the factor by which the ^{99}Tc^m thyroid image is multiplied so that the number of counts in the ^{99}Tc^m ROI are equal to those in the ^{201}Tl ROI.

6. The subtraction is carried out as follows:

Total ^{201}Tl counts $-$ (Total ^{99}Tc^m counts $\times$ CF)

This yields a 100% technetium subtraction. Further stepwise subtractions of 80, 60 and 40% can be easily computed by decreasing the value of the CF by the appropriate percentage.

9.6.8 TECHNIQUE (^{99}Tc^m INJECTION FIRST)

1. Ensure camera, film back and computer are set.
2. Position patient as described earlier and lock the trolley brakes. A head clamp may be used to prevent the patient from moving the head.
3. Store a marker view image for 30 s with the camera peaked on ^{57}Co, and mark the position of the markers on the persistence scope and the patient's skin for later reference. Remove the markers.
4. Set up the computer to record one frame per minute for 15 min. Peak the camera on ^{99}Tc^m.
5. Inject the patient intravenously with the measured dose of ^{99}Tc^m-pertechnetate and wait 60 s before starting acquisition.
   If the positioning is incorrect, then halt the acquisition, reposition and restart as soon as possible.
6. When acquisition is complete, without moving the patient, peak the camera on ^{201}Tl (30% window) and record a dynamic study of one frame per minute in a 64 × 64 word matrix for 5 min. This is the scatter image, which is necessary for correcting the crossover from ^{99}Tc^m into ^{201}Tl. Without this image the subtraction will be useless.
7. Following this acquisition, inject the patient intravenously with the measured dose of ^{201}Tl and wait 60 s before starting acquisition. Record at one frame per minute for 15 min.
8. When acquisition is complete, reposition the markers and record an image for 30 s as before. If the patient has moved significantly since the start of the study, this image can be used for movement correction if necessary during analysis.
9. Throughout the study, make sure the patient keeps still, otherwise the subtraction is useless.

9.6.9 ANALYSIS (^{99}Tc^m FIRST)

The analysis is essentially similar to the first technique, once the scatter image data are used to correct the ^{201}Tl data. Remember to normalize the data in terms of the different number of frames recorded, i.e. five frames of scatter compared to 15 frames of ^{201}Tl.

9.6.10 IMAGE LAYOUT

15 Multi ciné (^{201}Tl)	15 Multi ciné (^{201}Tl) Enhanced
0–15 min ^{201} Tl	0–15 min ^{99}Tc^{m}
^{201}Tl – ^{99}Tc^{m} Subtracted	^{201}Tl – ^{99}Tc^{m} Subtracted + enhanced

9.7 ADRENAL CORTEX IMAGING

9.7.1 PATIENT PREPARATION

Prior preparation with dexamethasone may be indicated in some patients. (Explain to the patient that the procedure involves two separate injections and four visits to the department.)

9.7.2 RADIOPHARMACEUTICALS AND DOSES

100 MBq ^{99}Tc^m-DMSA
8 MBq ^{75}Se-selenocholesterol

9.7.3 EQUIPMENT

The study is usually performed on a wide-field-of-view gamma camera fitted with a medium-energy collimator.

9.7.4 PATIENT POSITIONING

The patient is positioned prone on the imaging table, with the camera centred over the kidneys.

9.7.5 COMPUTER

All adrenal images are recorded on a computer using a 128 × 128 word matrix for 15 min per image.

   The marker images and the DMSA images are recorded for 30 s and 300 s, respectively, using 128 × 128 word matrices.

9.7.6 TECHNIQUE

1. The patient is injected IV with the measured dose of ^{99}Tc^m-DMSA and scanned 4 h later.
2. With the camera peaked on ^{99}Tc^m, the patient is positioned prone with the camera centred over the kidneys and a static image is stored on a 128 × 128 word matrix for 5 min duration. An analogue image is also recorded on film for the same time.
3. When the acquisition is complete, raise the camera (without any clockwise/anti-clockwise or forward/reverse movement) and, without moving the patient, locate the upper poles of the kidneys using a lead disc. Place a ^{57}Co marker at the upper pole of each kidney and lower the camera to its original position.

4. Peak the camera on ^{57}Co and record a 30 s set time image on the computer in a 128 × 128 word matrix. Record this image on film as well.

   Before removing the markers, outline their relative positions on the patient's back with indelible ink and tell the patient to get the marks renewed if they begin to fade.

5. Inject the patient with 8 MBq of Scintadren using a butterfly infusion set and flushing the dose through with a small volume of normal saline for injections. Do *not* draw blood back into the syringe as the dose may clot.

6. Arrange appointments with the patient for days 7, 9 and 14 following the injection.

7. On day 7 record a ^{75}Se uniformity correction image using all three peaks of ^{75}Se with the following window widths:

Low	120 keV	20%
Centre	140 keV	20%
Upper	270 keV	12%

8. Position patient as for day 0 and do the following:
   (a) Record at 15 min set time image in a 128 × 128 word matrix using triple peak settings.
   (b) When acquisition is complete, do not move the patient. Raise the camera and place the ^{57}Co markers on top of the marks on patient's back. Lower the camera to its original position. Peak the camera on ^{57}Co and store a 30 s image in a 128 × 128 matrix.

   In both instances, record analogue images for the same length of time.

9. Repeat steps 7 and 8 on day 9 and day 14.

10. On the final day of the study, it may be necessary to perform a liver–spleen scan using ^{99}Tc^{m}-colloid, for subtraction and localization.

9.7.7 ANALYSIS

1. The DMSA image is analysed using the standard DMSA analyses to obtain divided renal function values.

2. Images of ^{75}Se are recorded with and without the ^{57}Co markers superimposed.

3. Images of ^{75}Se pictures are also recorded with and without the renal DMSA image overlaid.

4. The DMSA analysis program may be used to analyse the adrenal images from each day of the study, to determine the divided function.

5. The percentage of the injected dose taken up by each adrenal gland may also be calculated, provided the syringe data are recorded on the computer prior to the injection. The same calculation as that used to measure thyroid uptake may be used if depth correction is not to be applied.

9.8 ^{131}I-MIBG PHAEOCHROMOCYTOMA IMAGING

9.8.1 PATIENT PREPARATION

The patient is given Lugol's solution (40 mg iodide) 6 drops per day before and for 4 days after the IV injection of MIBG.

9.8.2 RADIOPHARMACEUTICAL AND DOSE

18 MBq/1.73 m^2 ^{131}I-MIBG
100 MBq ^{99}Tc^m-DMSA

9.8.3 EQUIPMENT

The study is performed on a wide-field-of-view gamma camera fitted with a medium-energy collimator.

9.8.4 PATIENT POSITIONING

The patient is positioned prone for the posterior views and supine for the anterior views on the imaging table.

9.8.5 COMPUTER

All MIBG images are recorded for 10 min per view using a 128 × 128 word matrix.
   The ^{99}Tc^m-DMSA image is recorded for 5 min and the corresponding ^{57}Co marker view is recorded for 30 s duration.

9.8.6 TECHNIQUE

1. The patient is injected IV with the measured dose of ^{99}Tc^m-DMSA and scanned 4 h later.
2. With the camera peaked on ^{99}Tc^m, the patient is positioned prone with the camera centred over the kidneys and a static image is stored in a 128 × 128 matrix. An analogue image is also recorded on film for the same time.
3. When the acquisition is complete, raise the camera (without any clockwise/anti-clockwise or forward/reverse movement) and, without moving the patient, locate the upper poles of the kidneys using a lead disc. Place a ^{57}Co marker at the upper pole of each kidney and lower the camera to its original position.

4. Peak the camera on ^{57}Co and acquire a 30 s set time image on the computer in a 128 × 128 word matrix. Record this image on film as well.

   Before removing the markers, outline their positions on the patient's back with indelible ink and tell the patient to get the marks renewed if they begin to fade.
5. Inject the patient with the dose of ^{131}I-MIBG, slowly over a period of 5–10 min, and monitor the patient for any reactions. Record the BP and pulse every minute for the duration of the injection.
6. The following set of images are recorded at 24 h after injection: anterior head and chest, anterior abdomen, anterior pelvis, posterior head and chest and posterior abdomen for 10 min per image.

   A posterior abdomen view with ^{57}Co markers is also recorded for 30 s with the camera peaked on ^{57}Co.
7. The imaging procedure is repeated at 72 h and 7 days after injection, if indicated.

9.9 TESTICULAR IMAGING

9.9.1 PATIENT PREPARATION

None.

9.9.2 RADIOPHARMACEUTICAL AND DOSE

500 MBq of ^{99}Tc^m-pertechnetate

This is the adult dose and should be adjusted in children in relation to body surface area. Also 400 mg of potassium perchlorate (2 × 200 mg tablets) is given orally to block the thyroid. This is the adult dose and should be adjusted in children in relation to body surface area.

9.9.3 EQUIPMENT

A standard-field camera with a converging collimator is used. Any other camera may be used provided the data system has some form of hardware or software zoom.

9.9.4 PATIENT POSITIONING

The patient is positioned supine on the imaging table, with legs abducted, the scrotal area parallel to the collimator supported by towels, with the penis taped back over the pubis with micropore tape. The collimator is centred over the median raphe. A piece of lead apron is placed over the thighs and under the scrotum to reduce the soft-tissue background.

9.9.5 COMPUTER

The computer is set up to record the dynamic phase of the study at one frame per second for 40 s using a 64 × 64 byte matrix. The static images are recorded using a 128 × 128 word matrix.

9.9.6 TECHNIQUE

1. The patient is given the perchlorate tablets and positioned as described under patient positioning. It is necessary to use markers and the persistence monitor to achieve accurate positioning.
2. Ensure camera and film back are set.
3. Ensure computer is set.

4. Give bolus injection of pertechnetate, starting camera and computer at moment of cuff release.
5. Record a vascular phase image on film for 30 s following cuff release.
6. Record two further images for 700 000 counts each, with the camera intensity slightly reduced. Back them up on a data system using a 128 × 128 word matrix.

9.9.7 IMAGE LAYOUT

0–30 s	Image 1 700 000
Image 2 700 000	

9.10 TRH TEST

9.10.1 PATIENT PREPARATION

The patient should be warned regarding the possible short-term side effects of the TRH.

9.10.2 PHARMACEUTICAL AND DOSE

0.2 mg/2 ml Protirelin (TRH – Roche)

9.10.3 TECHNIQUE

1. Take a 10 ml baseline blood sample in a plain glass tube (for clotted blood).
2. Inject the dose of TRH slowly through the same needle.
3. Take further 10 ml clotted blood samples at 20 min and 60 min.
4. Send all the samples to the laboratory for TSH level estimation.

9.11 CALCITONIN PROVOCATION TEST

9.11.1 PATIENT PREPARATION

The patient should be fasted from midnight.

If pentagastrin is used, the patient should be warned about the unpleasant side effects, e.g. nausea, epigastric or chest tightness, which lasts about 2–3 min.

With whisky, the amount used may make the patient drunk, and the patient may thus not be allowed home until the effect is over.

Check that the patient is not driving after the test.

9.11.2 PHARMACEUTICAL AND DOSE

Pentagastrin 0.5 μg/kg
Whisky 50 ml (pharmacy)

9.11.3 TECHNIQUE

1. Check that the patient has fasted overnight.
2. Check that the centrifuge is cooled to 4°C to separate the plasma immediately after the test is over.
3. Ensure you have three heparin (orange) bottles cooled in a beaker of ice to receive the blood samples.

Pentagastrin test

1. Take a 10 ml basal blood sample.
2. Slowly inject the pentagastrin IV.
3. Take 10 ml blood samples at 2 and 5 min.

Whisky test

1. Take the 10 ml basal blood sample.
2. Give the oral dose of whisky.
3. Take 10 ml blood samples at 5 and 10 min.

Note
The blood samples should be centrifuged at 4°C immediately after the test is completed and stored for calcitonin assay.

CHAPTER TEN

HAEMATOLOGY STUDIES

INTRODUCTION

Red blood cells may be labelled with ^{51}Cr in the form of sodium chromate. The binding of ^{51}Cr to the red cells is very tight and if these labelled red cells are injected into the body intravenously, most of the ^{51}Cr remains bound to the cells until they are destroyed. The labelling procedure must be carried out carefully so that no significant damage occurs to the red cells.

By reinjecting a known volume of the patient's own red blood cells labelled with a known amount of ^{51}Cr and measuring the activity in a second sample of blood after allowing a suitable period for mixing, all of the information necessary to calculate red cell volume is available. In terms of patient preparation, it is important that blood should neither be given nor lost while the test is being conducted, otherwise falsely reduced or elevated values will be obtained.

Red cell survival studies are used to assess haemolysis in patients with anaemia of unknown aetiology. If the time pattern of the radioactivity in the blood is followed over several days, a measure of the life span of the red cells in the body is obtained. The period usually determined is the time of the radioactivity to fall to one half of its original level.

The major site of removal of damaged red blood cells is the spleen. In the splenic sequestration study the ^{51}Cr released from disintegrating red cells also accumulates in the liver. The ratio of the spleen to liver ^{51}Cr activity, monitored by surface counting over several days, provides a rough measure of the degree of hypersplenism, and may indicate the value of splenectomy as therapy.

Plasma volume is measured using the same principle as the red cell mass, but using ^{125}I-human serum albumin.

^{111}In-labelled white cell imaging is now a common procedure in all well-equipped nuclear medicine centres. It is used for the detection and localization of acute inflammations such as cellulitis and abscesses. ^{111}In-labelled white cell imaging is preferred for localizing intraabdominal abscesses because of the lack of gastrointestinal uptake seen on ^{67}Ga images. The results are also more quickly available (at 24 h) than with gallium.

Gastrointestinal blood loss is measured using the patient's own red blood cells labelled with ^{51}Cr to estimate accurately the quantity of red cells lost through GI bleeding.

10.1 RADIOPHARMACEUTICALS

10.1.1 ^{51}Cr-RBCs

> **Note**
> *Aseptic procedure*   Switch on the microbiological safety cabinet at least 5 min before starting.

1. Collect the following:
   (a) five 20 ml syringes
   (b) one 1 ml syringe
   (c) three 21G (green) needles
   (d) three 5 inch filling tubes (kwills)
   (e) ^{51}Cr-sodium chromate (37 MBq/ml)
   (f) four 10 ml ampoules Sodium Chloride Injection BP 0.9 w/v
   (g) 1.5 ml ACD solution (USP solution A) which comes in a pred-ispensed vial
2. Using a 20 ml syringe with a green needle, draw 15 ml of blood from the patient with a clean venepuncture, and transfer the blood to the ACD solution in the safety cabinet. Gently rotate the tube to mix thoroughly.
3. Centrifuge the bottle for 15 min at 1300g. Remember the *balance* tube.
4. After centrifuging, spray the bottle with chlorhexidine in spirit and transfer to the safety cabinet without disturbing the packed red blood cells. Assemble a 20 ml syringe and kwill. Draw off the plasma as completely as possible, avoiding any red cells. Discard the plasma into the sluice and flush.
5. Add the appropriate activity of ^{51}Cr-sodium chromate solution (1.5 MBq for red-cell mass, 3 MBq for red-cell survival) using a 1 ml syringe and green needle. If the volume of ^{51}Cr-sodium chromate solution is less than 0.2 ml, dilute to 0.2 ml in the syringe with Sodium Chloride Injection BP 0.9% w/v.
6. Allow to stand in the cabinet for 15 min, mixing gently by rotation every 5 min.
7. Wash the cells with Sodium Chloride Injection BP 0.9% w/v as follows:
   (a) Add Sodium Chloride Injection BP 0.9% w/v to fill the bottle (up to 20 ml) and mix gently by rotation.
   (b) Centrifuge for 10 min at 1300g. Remember the *balance* bottle!
   (c) Transfer the bottle back to the safety cabinet, after spraying with chlorhexidine. Assemble a 20 ml syringe and kwill. Draw off the

saline wash as completely as possible, avoiding any red cells. Discard the wash into the sluice and flush.

8. Repeat the saline wash as above.
9. Resuspend the cells with Sodium Chloride Injection BP 0.9% w/v to fill the bottle (up to 20 ml) and mix gently by rotation.
10. Label the vial with activity, volume, time, date, batch number and patient's name, and prepare two further identical labels, one for the record book and one for the patient's request form.
11. Complete a sheet in the blood products records book, including the following:
    (a) date
    (b) name of preparation
    (c) lot number of ACD solution
    (d) lot number of Sodium Chloride Injection BP 0.9% w/v
    (e) lot number of the ^{51}Cr-sodium chromate
    (f) time
    (g) batch number
    (h) technician's initials
12. Attach a specimen label to the record sheet.

10.2 RED-CELL MASS ESTIMATION

10.2.1 PROCEDURE

1. Record the patient's height (cm) and weight (kg) on the patient's request form.
2. Label the patient's red blood cells as described above.
3. Using a 20 ml syringe, accurately draw up 16 ml of the labelled cells and inject *intravenously* into the patient. Save the rest for preparing the standard.
4. At 10 min after injection, take a 10 ml blood sample from the opposite arm into which the cells were injected. Put 4 ml of this blood into a (pink) EDTA tube. Send it to haematology for a PCV (packed cell volume) estimation. Put 3 ml blood into each of two more (pink) EDTA tubes. Add a knifepoint of saponin powder to each and mix them on a rotary mixer for 5 min.
5. At 20 min after injection, take a 6 ml blood sample from the opposite arm into which the cells were injected. Put 3 ml blood into each of two more (pink) EDTA tubes. Add a knifepoint of saponin powder to each and mix them on a rotary mixer for 5 min.
6. To prepare the standard, add a knifepoint of saponin powder to the residual labelled cells and mix them on the rotary mixer for 5 min using a graduated glass pipette, pipette 1 ml of the mixed red cells into a volumetric flask and make up to 100 ml with distilled water and mix thoroughly.
7. To prepare samples for counting, using separate graduated glass pipettes:
   (a) Pipette a 3 ml sample from the 10 min blood samples into a large Luckham's (10 ml) tube.
   (b) Pipette a 3 ml sample from the 20 min blood samples into a large Luckham's (10 ml) tube.
   (c) Pipette a 3 ml sample from the standard into a large Luckham's (10 ml) tube.
8. Count these samples and a background sample for 1000 s each on the ^{51}Cr window using a suitable gamma counter.
9. Plot the 10 and 20 min sample counts (minus background) against time on semi-log graph paper and extrapolate to zero to obtain counts at zero time.

10.2.2 CALCULATIONS

Perform the following calculations:

Red-cell volume, RCV $= \dfrac{S \times D \times V \times Hv}{B}$

where S = counts per minute per millilitre of standard, D = dilution of standard, V = volume injected, Hv = PCV ÷ 100 and B = counts per minute per milliltre of blood at time 0.

Plasma volume $= \dfrac{RCV\ (100 - H)}{H}$

where $H = 0.91 \times$ PCV.

Normal ranges for red-cell volumes are: male, 25–35 ml/kg; female, 20–30 ml/kg. Estimated plasma volume is approximately 40 ml/kg.

10.3 RED-CELL SURVIVAL AND SEQUESTRATION STUDIES

10.3.1 RED-CELL SURVIVAL

Patient preparation

The patient should not have a blood transfusion once the study commences. If the patient is subject to repeated blood transfusions, then the study should be coordinated to begin soon after a blood transfusion has been given.

Procedure

Label the patient's red cells with 3 MBq of ^{51}Cr-sodium chromate as described in section 10.1.1. Using a 20 ml syringe, accurately draw up 16 ml of the labelled cells and inject intravenously into the patient. Save the rest for preparing the standard.

Daily

Take a 12 ml sample of blood from the patient (from the opposite arm to the one which had the labelled cells injected), and put 4 ml into each of three (pink) EDTA tubes. Send one of these to haematology for a PCV estimation. To each of the other two, add a knifepoint of saponin powder and mix the samples on a rotary mixer for 5 min. Pipette a 5 ml sample from these two into a counting tube. If a 5 ml aliquot cannot be obtained, the sample volume should be made up to 5 ml with deionized water and the counts corrected for this, later.

> **Note**
> For patients on dialysis, the blood samples should be taken *before* dialysis commences.

This daily sampling should be continued until the counts of the last sample are half those of the first sample.

To prepare the standard

Add a knifepoint of saponin to the residual labelled cells and mix well. Pipette 1 ml into a volumetric flask and make up to 100 ml with deionized water. Pipette 5 ml of this into a counting tube.

Counting

Count the last blood sample taken, for 10 000 counts on the ^{51}Cr window. Note the time taken, and count all the samples and the standard for this length of time.

Calculations

1. Calculate the red-cell mass as in Section 10.2.2.
2. Correct the sample counts for background.
3. Correct the counts for PCV by multiplying the counts for each day by

$$\frac{\text{PCV for day 0}}{\text{PCV for each day}}$$

4. Express the counts from each sample as a percentage of the counts at day 0, i.e.

$$\frac{\text{Counts}}{\text{Counts on day 0}} \times 100$$

Table 10.1

Day	Correction factor
0	1.00
1	1.01
2	1.03
3	1.04
4	1.06
5	1.07
6	1.08
7	1.10
8	1.11
9	1.13
10	1.14
11	1.16
12	1.17
13	1.19
14	1.20
15	1.21
16	1.23
17	1.24
18	1.26
19	1.27
20	1.29
21	1.31
22	1.32
23	1.34
24	1.35
25	1.37
26	1.38
27	1.40
28	1.41
29	1.43
30	1.44

Plot these counts against time on semi-log graph paper and read off the time for 50% counts. The normal range is 25–35 days.

5. Correct the counts for elution of the ^{51}Cr from the red cells by multiplying each day's counts by the correction factor for that day as given in Table 10.1.

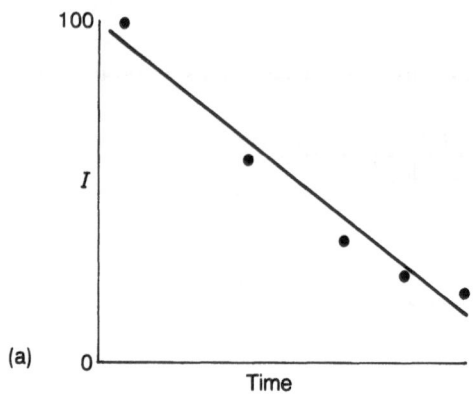

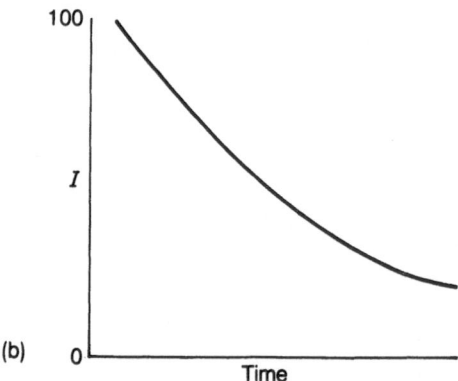

Fig. 10.1 Time–activity curves for red-cell survival study: (a) gradient 7.4, intercept 102, correlation coefficient 1.0, mean life 12.8, half-life 6.4; (b) correlation coefficient 1.0, mean life 5.6, half-life 3.6.

6. Plot the counts against time on linear graph paper. If the points lie close to a straight line, read off the mean red-cell life. This is the time taken to reach zero counts, i.e. the intercept of the fitted line with the time axis $(Y = 0)$.

If the linear fit is not acceptable, then try plotting counts against time on semi-log graph paper (Fig. 10.1). If the points lie close to a straight line, then read off the mean red-cell life. This is the time taken to reach 37.5% of counts at zero time. The normal range for mean red-cell life is 120 ± 14 days.

10.3.2 RED-CELL SEQUESTRATION

Patient preparation

Ideally the patient should not have a blood transfusion once the study commences. If the patient is subject to repeated blood transfusions, then the study should be coordinated to begin soon after a blood transfusion has been given. If the patient has a blood transfusion in the middle of the study, this should be noted.

Technique

At least 24 h before the sequestration study is started, the patient has a liver–spleen scan performed to assess splenic size and to outline the areas for counting. It is recommended that the liver–spleen study be performed on Friday and the sequestration study commenced on the following Monday.

The areas for counting are marked following the injection of the $^{99}Tc^m$-colloid, using a lead disc of appropriate size roughly corresponding to the diameter of the scintillation detector.

The early blood pool phase (i.e. at 1 min following injection) is used to outline the heart accurately. For marking, the patient is positioned supine under the camera and with the camera pointing down, collimator face parallel to the floor. The lead disc is placed over the patient's heart blood pool and by visually monitoring the persistence scope image, the disc is positioned so that it is well clear of the liver and spleen. The counting site is marked using indelible ink by tracing along the edge of the disc.

At 20 min after injection the liver and spleen are similarly marked. The spleen is generally better visualized on the posterior view, with the patient lying prone under the camera.

Note
It is important that the patient's heart, liver and spleen are marked with the patient lying in the same position as for the subsequent counting.

At least 24 h later the patient's red blood cells are labelled with 3 MBq ^{51}Cr-sodium chromate as described in section 10.1.1 and the procedure for red-cell mass is carried out.

To prepare the standard

Add a knifepoint of saponin powder to the residual labelled cells and mix well. Pipette 1 ml into a volumetric flask and make up to 100 ml with deionized water. Pipette a 5 ml aliquot of this into a counting tube narrow enough to fit into the well of the surface counting probe. (The volume may need to be reduced to ensure that the liquid level is well below the top surface of the well in the detector).

Daily counting

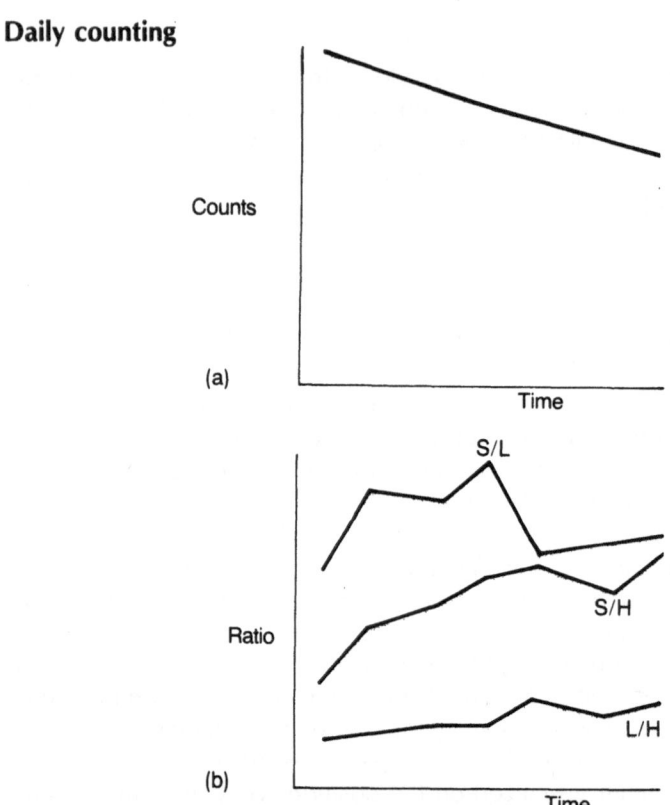

Fig. 10.2 Time–activity curves for red-cell sequestration study: (a) half-life 27.7 days (correct value 28 days); (b) spleen to liver (S/L) ratio, spleen to heart (S/H) ratio, liver to heart (L/H) ratio.

Switch on the counter at least 30 min before use, and peak the counter using the standard. Position the detector vertical, ensuring that it is in contact with the patient's skin.

Count the three sites (heart, liver and spleen), the background and the standard for 300 s each. Ensure that the patient does not move during the counting period.

Plot the standard counts against time on semi-log paper (Fig. 10.2a) and check that they lie on a straight line ($T_{1/2}$ = 27.8 days).

The surface counting is continued for approximately 4–6 weeks and the patient attends daily for the first week and every other day for the duration of the study. The duration of the study will depend on the red-cell survival time.

Calculations

Calculate and plot the following ratios against time on linear graph paper (Fig. 10.2b):

$$\frac{\text{Spleen}}{\text{Heart}} \qquad \frac{\text{Liver}}{\text{Heart}} \qquad \frac{\text{Spleen}}{\text{Liver}}$$

10.4 ^{51}Cr GASTROINTESTINAL BLOOD LOSS STUDY

10.4.1 PATIENT PREPARATION

There is no patient preparation.

10.4.2 METHOD

1. Label the patient's red blood cells with approximately 5 MBq ^{51}Cr-sodium chromate using the procedure described in Section 10.1.1.
2. Inject 10 ml of the labelled cells intravenously.
3. Instruct the ward to collect 24 h stool samples for at least 7 days. Provide the ward with (2 l capacity) containers, lids and instructions. See instruction sheet in Table 10.2.
4. Take a 10 ml blood sample into a lithium heparin sample tube every 2 or 3 days.

Table 10.2 Typical instruction sheet for ^{51}Cr GI blood loss study.

Department of Nuclear Medicine

Gastrointestinal blood loss estimation

Surname	Unit no.
First name	Sex
Date of birth	Consultant
Address	Ward/clinic

Instructions
Daily stool collections for the next 5 days, i.e.

From   to

1. Please put each 24 h stool collections into the containers provided. *No urine please.*
2. Dilute and add 1 litre of preservative concentrate (provided) to each container and *seal well*. Instructions for diluting the preservative are on the container. *Do not add anything else* (i.e. toilet paper, polythene bags, etc.).
3. Label each container with the patient's name and the date of collection, using a waterproof marker pen. If labels are to be used, then please make sure that they do not fall off.
4. As soon as the 5 day collection is complete, send all the containers and the empty preservative containers to the Nuclear Medicine Dept.
5. If there are any queries, please ring the Nuclear Medicine Dept:
   ext.   and ask for

10.4.3 COUNTING

1. At the end of the week when all the samples are collected, homogenize the faecal samples (e.g. by using a paint can shaker).
2. Add the 10 ml blood samples to independent containers containing 1 litre of deionized water, and shake well.
3. Count all the samples, faecal and blood, using a large scintillation detector with the counter set to detect ^{51}Cr for 30 min per sample.

10.4.4 CALCULATIONS

Plot the counts from the 10 ml blood samples against time on semi-log paper and determine the appropriate counts for each day of the study, by interpolating where necessary. Calculate the following:

$$\text{Faecal blood loss} = \frac{\text{Counts per minute in faecal specimen} \times 10}{\text{Counts per minute in 10 ml of blood sample}}$$

The result is expressed in millilitres of blood.

10.5 PLASMA VOLUME ESTIMATION USING ^{125}I-HSA

Iodinated ^{125}I-HSA is used to measure plasma volume. Iodination of the albumin molecule does not alter its biological properties. Once the protein is metabolized, part of the iodine is excreted and a certain amount is retained by the thyroid.

The rate of disappearance of albumin from the blood is approximately 7–10% per hour. This loss can be neglected during the 10–15 min mixing interval except in pathological conditions when the rate of loss can reach 30% per hour. Therefore, the tracer concentration should be determined before it leaves the circulation by taking at least two blood samples at different time intervals and extrapolating back to obtain the zero time concentration.

Iodinated protein tends to stick to glass and polythene and therefore when preparing the standard the diluent should be a solution of albumin (1% aqueous) or a detergent, not water.

10.5.1 PATIENT PREPARATION

Nil.

10.5.2 METHOD

1. Weigh the patient and record the weight on the patient's request form.
2. Take a 10 ml background blood sample and put it in a lithium heparin sample tube.
3. Inject 0.004 MBq/kg ^{125}I-HSA.
4. Take 10 ml blood samples from the patient's opposite arm at 10 and 20 min after injection and put into lithium heparin tubes.
5. Take a 5 ml blood sample and put it in a pink (EDTA) tube and send to haematology for a packed cell volume (PCV) estimation.
6. Prepare a standard with a 1:100 dilution, using a 1% aqueous solution of human serum albumin as diluent.
7. Centrifuge and pipette 5 ml aliquots of plasma from each of the samples using separate glass pipettes. Pipette off a 5 ml sample of the standard using a separate pipette. Count all the samples together and a background using the gamma counter set to count ^{125}I so that at least 10 000 counts are obtained from the 20 min sample.

10.5.3 CALCULATIONS

Plot the background-corrected counts against time on semi-log graph paper and obtain the plasma counts at zero time by extrapolating back to zero time:

$$\text{Plasma volume} = \frac{S \times V \times D}{B}$$

where S = standard counts per minute less background, V = volume injected, D = dilution of standard, and B = counts at time 0 less background. The result is expressed in millilitres per kilogram body weight. The normal range is 31–55 ml/kg for an adult male and 36–50 ml/kg for an adult female.

10.6 ^{111}In LEUCOCYTE IMAGING STUDY

10.6.1 PATIENT PREPARATION

Nil.

10.6.2 RADIOPHARMACEUTICAL AND DOSE

18 MBq ^{111}In-labelled autologous leucocytes

10.6.3 PATIENT POSITIONING

The patient is positioned supine on the imaging table for the anterior views and prone for the posterior views (Fig. 10.3). The camera is only placed under the imaging table if the patient is unable to lie prone.

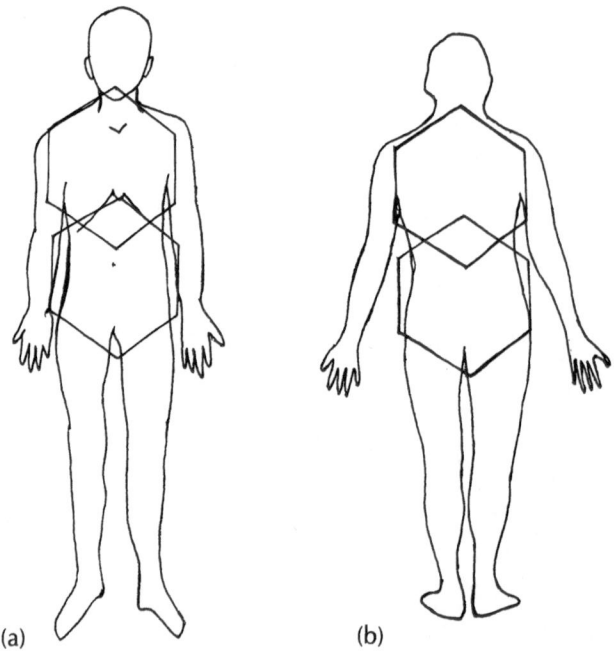

(a)   (b)

Fig. 10.3 Patient positioning for a leucocyte imaging study: (a) anterior; (b) posterior.

10.6.4 EQUIPMENT

A wide-field-of-view gamma camera is used, fitted with a medium-energy collimator and equipped with analyser facility to sum up the counts from the two main photopeaks of ¹¹¹In.

10.6.5 COMPUTER

The computer is set up to record static images in a 128 × 128 word matrix for 7 min per view. If a single view only needs to be done, then this should be recorded for 15 min per view using 256 × 256 matrix.

10.6.6 TECHNIQUE

1. Using an aseptic technique, take 60 ml of blood from the patient using an 18G needle into a 60 ml syringe containing 500 i.u. of preservative-free heparin.
2. Label the white cells with ¹¹¹In-oxine. (It is beyond the scope of this book to describe a white-cell labelling technique in detail. However, a well tried technique is presented in diagrammatic form (Fig. 10.4).
3. Reinject the labelled cells into the same patient and wait 2 h.
4. Position patient as in patient positioning.
5. Ensure camera and computer are set.
6. Following the image layout below, record anterior chest, anterior abdomen and pelvis, posterior chest and posterior abdomen and pelvis, for 7 min per view, ensuring slight overlap between the views.
7. Repeat the necessary view(s) at approximately 24 h after injection. Lateral or oblique views may also need to be done if clinically indicated.

10.6.7 IMAGE LAYOUT

Anterior Chest and abdomen	Posterior Chest and abdomen
Anterior Abdomen and pelvis	Posterior Abdomen and pelvis

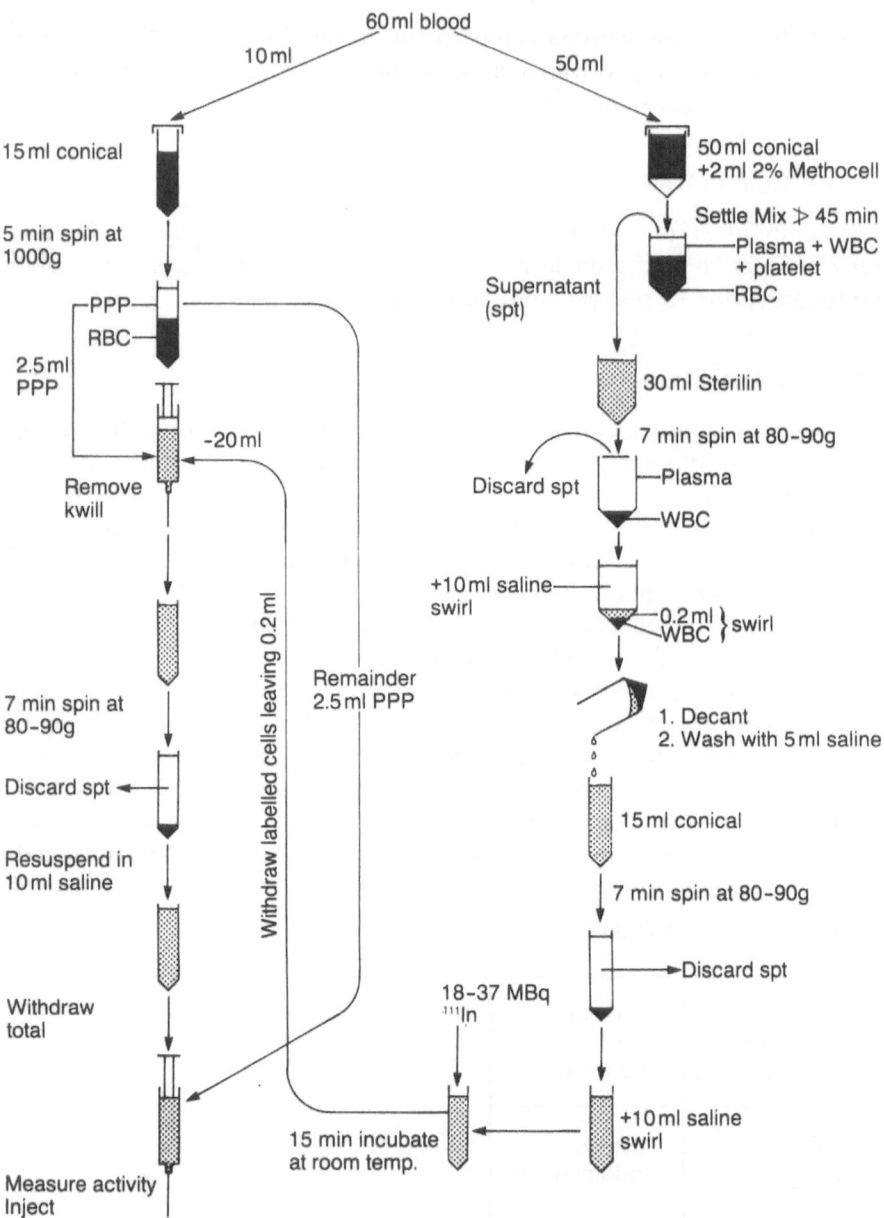

Fig. 10.4 Preparation of ¹¹¹In-leucocytes: a well tried white-cell labelling technique. This procedure *must* be carried out in a microbiological safety cabinet, class II.

CHAPTER ELEVEN

MISCELLANEOUS STUDIES .

INTRODUCTION

^{67}Ga imaging currently remains the most established nuclear medicine procedure for localizing soft tissue tumours and inflammatory processes. It is used routinely for the diagnosis, evaluation and follow-up of lymphomas and inflammatory processes although the mechanism of gallium uptake in these conditions is not entirely clear. For diagnosing intraabdominal abscesses, ^{111}In-labelled white cells should be used since gallium is excreted into the bowel and because the resultant high background may disguise other lesions. Liver–spleen subtraction imaging has been found to be useful in patients suspected of intrahepatic abscesses. The target-to-background ratio increases with time so that imaging on successive days improves detection of the lesions.

Epiphora is a fairly common ophthalmic problem caused by the blockage of the normal pathway of drainage of tears from the eye into the nasopharynx. By placing a drop of ^{99}Tc^{m}-tin colloid in the eye and recording a series of sequential images, it is possible to image the flow of tears through the nasolacrimal drainage system. The technique is simple, safe and much more physiologic than other techniques available for diagnosing the potency of the lacrimal drainage apparatus.

There are certain benign and malignant lesions that leak protein into the GI tract. These lesions are rare and protein loss through this route is difficult to quantitate. ^{51}Cr-chromic chloride is used to determine quantitatively whether an excessive amount of protein is lost in the GI tract.

11.1 RADIOPHARMACEUTICALS

11.1.1 ^{67}Ga CITRATE

This is received ready for use and the only procedure necessary is to check the total activity in the vial against the label and the expiry date.

1. Prepare a fresh sheet in the ^{67}Ga citrate record book, noting the following:
   (a) date
   (b) time of activity measured
   (c) batch number
   (d) expiry date
   (e) signature
   (f) total activity in vial
   (g) manufacturer's lot number and expiry date
2. Doses should be withdrawn aseptically in a laminar flow cabinet, and the syringe fitted with a blue (23G) needle and syringe shield, ready for injection.
3. Record the following in the ^{67}Ga citrate record book:
   (a) date of dose withdrawal
   (b) dose and volume withdrawn
   (c) patient's name and weight
4. Attach a specimen label to the record sheet showing the activity, volume, time, date, expiry, patient's name and batch number.

11.2 ^{67}Ga IMAGING

11.2.1 PATIENT PREPARATION

Oral laxatives are given to the patient, to be taken every evening starting on the day of ^{67}Ga injection and to continue until the last day of imaging.

The very young and patients with diarrhoea must *not* be given laxatives.

11.2.2 RADIOPHARMACEUTICAL AND DOSE

1.85 MBq/kg ^{67}Ga citrate injected IV

11.2.3 PATIENT POSITIONING

The patient is positioned supine on the imaging table, with the camera above for the anterior views and prone for the posterior views. The camera is only placed under the table if the patient is unable to lie prone.

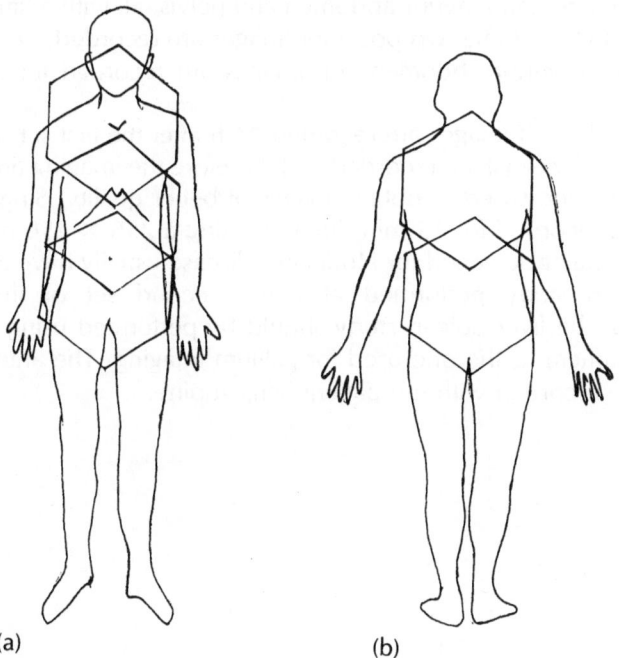

(a)   (b)

Fig. 11.1 Patient positioning for a ^{67}Ga citrate imaging study: (a) anterior; (b) posterior.

11.2.4 EQUIPMENT

A wide-field-of-view gamma camera fitted with a medium- or high-energy collimator is used. The camera should ideally be capable of accumulating counts from the three main photopeaks of ^{67}Ga using 20% windows.

11.2.5 COMPUTER

Normally a computer is only used if liver–spleen subtraction is to be carried out, but it can be used for backing up the studies. The images should be recorded using a 128 × 128 word matrix.

11.2.6 TECHNIQUE

1. The patient is injected intravenously with the measured dose of ^{67}Ga citrate and instructed to take the laxatives, i.e. one or two capsules to be taken every night.
2. The first set of images are recorded after 48 or 72 h depending on whether the patient is injected on Friday or Monday.

   The images recorded are anterior head, neck and chest, anterior chest and abdomen, and anterior abdomen and pelvis, all with a little overlap between images. Only two posterior images are recorded, i.e. posterior chest and posterior abdomen. All images are recorded for 300 s per view.
3. The second set of images are recorded 24 h after the first set. Generally only selected view(s) are recorded and therefore the imaging time can be substantially increased to obtain images of better quality. Single images should be recorded for 15 min duration using a 256 × 256 matrix.

   Patients being screened for Hodgkin's disease usually have a standard liver–spleen study performed after the second set of imaging. If requested, the liver–spleen study should be performed using the same gamma camera as the one used for gallium imaging. The anterior view should be recorded with the patient lying supine.

11.2.7 IMAGE LAYOUT

Anterior Head, neck and chest	
Anterior Chest and abdomen	Posterior Chest and abdomen
Anterior Abdomen and pelvis	Posterior Abdomen and pelvis

11.2.8 LIVER–SPLEEN SUBTRACTION

In some patients, liver–spleen subtraction may need to be performed. The procedure is as follows:

Record the anterior abdomen view (^{67}Ga) last, making sure that the liver is clearly within the field of view.

Then, without moving the patient, inject ^{99}Tc^m-tin colloid for liver–spleen imaging and leave the patient in the same position for 15 min. It is critical that the patient does *not* move during this waiting period, if the subtraction is to be successful.

At the end of this period, peak the camera on ^{99}Tc^m and record the liver–spleen image (using the same matrix size as the corresponding gallium image) for 500 000 counts.

The subtraction is carried out as follows:

1. Select the ^{99}Tc^m-tin colloid image and carefully outline the liver using an irregular region of interest. Note the total counts within this region (TC).
2. Recall the corresponding ^{67}Ga image and overlay the region outlined on the ^{99}Tc^m liver–spleen image and note the total number of counts within the region (GA).
3. Correct the ^{99}Tc^m image for the difference in counts, i.e. multiply the ^{99}Tc^m image by the factor GA ÷ TC, so that the counts in the ^{99}Tc^m image will match the counts in the ^{67}Ga liver region.
4. Subtract this fraction of the ^{99}Tc^m liver matrix from the ^{67}Ga matrix, i.e.

$${}^{67}\text{Ga} - [(\text{GA} \div \text{TC}) \times \text{TC}]$$

where TC = total counts from ^{99}Tc^m liver image and GA = total counts from ^{67}Ga liver region.

11.3 LACRIMAL SCINTIGRAPHIC IMAGING

11.3.1 PATIENT PREPARATION

Soft or hard contact lenses must be removed. Explain procedure to the patient.

11.3.2 RADIOPHARMACEUTICAL AND DOSE

1 MBq ^{99}Tc^m-tin colloid

Dilute the ^{99}Tc^m-colloid with sodium chloride for injections 0.9% w/v to give a concentration of approximately 83 MBq/ml (equivalent to 1 MBq in a 12 μl drop).

This radiopharmaceutical is chosen because its pH is acceptable to the eye and its viscosity is slightly higher than pertechnetate. Pertechnetate would also get absorbed into the intraocular spaces, increasing the radiation dose to the lens.

11.3.3 PATIENT POSITIONING

The patient is positioned sitting with the chin on a chin rest if using a pinhole collimator.

If using a higher-resolution collimator, then the patient sits with the forehead firmly against the collimator.

11.3.4 EQUIPMENT

Any gamma camera may be used fitted with a pinhole, snout or high-resolution collimator.

A suitable chin rest as used by ophthalmologists is most useful for patient comfort.

11.3.5 COMPUTER

The computer is set up to record one frame every minute for 12 min in a 64 × 64 word matrix.

11.3.6 TECHNIQUE

1. Explain the procedure to the patient.

2. Position patient at the correct distance using ^{57}Co marker sources so that the field of view covers both eyes, including the outer canthus and the nose.

   If quantitation is to be performed, then attach a marker source to the patient's forehead, just above the nasion.
3. Using suitable dropper devices, instil the radiopharmaceutical in each eye simultaneously, as follows:

Instillation procedure

> **Note**
> If the patient's eye(s) are watering, dab them dry before proceeding.

(a) Ask the patient to tilt head back and, with eyes wide open, look upwards.
(b) Pull down the lower eyelids, enough to form a pouch and *carefully* instil the drop in each eye.
(c) Immediately position the patient as described above. Velcro bands may be used for restraining to minimize patient movement.
(d) Start the computer and camera recording as soon as the patient is in position.
(e) If the patient's eye(s) begin to water, then dab them dry gently with tissue paper.

If indicated, a single delayed image should be recorded at 30 min. Record it for 1 min on a 64 × 64 word matrix, as a one frame dynamic to maintain continuity with the initial images. If there is evidence of obstruction, the eyes should be washed out using saline eye wash.

11.3.7 IMAGE LAYOUT

1 min	3 min
5 min	7 min
9 min	12 min

11.4 GASTROINTESTINAL PROTEIN LOSS ESTIMATION USING ^{51}Cr-CHROMIC CHLORIDE

11.4.1 PATIENT PREPARATION

Nil.

11.4.2 RADIOPHARMACEUTICAL AND DOSE

Approximately 0.3 MBq of ^{51}Cr-chromic chloride in 5 ml

11.4.3 PROCEDURE

1. Dilute 1 MBq of ^{51}Cr-chromic chloride to 12.5 ml with 0.9% w/v sodium chloride for injections using an aseptic technique.

Table 11.1 Typical instruction sheet for ^{51}Cr GI protein loss study.

Department of Nuclear Medicine

Protein losing enteropathy

Surname	Unit no.
First name	Sex
Date of birth	Consultant
Address	Ward/clinic

Instructions
Daily stool collections for the next 5 days, i.e.

from   to

1. Please put each 24 h stool collections into the containers provided. *No urine please.*
2. Dilute and add 1 litre of the preservative fluid (provided) to each container and *seal well.* Instructions for diluting the preservative are on the container.
    Please do not add anything else (i.e. toilet paper, polythene bags, etc.).
3. Label each container with the patient's name and the date of collection, using a waterproof marker pen. If labels are to be used, then please make sure that they do not fall off.
4. As soon as the 5 day collection is complete, send all the containers and the empty preservative containers to the Nuclear Medicine Dept.
5. If there are any queries, please ring the Nuclear Medicine Dept:

    ext.   and ask for

2. Inject 5 ml of this diluted ^{51}Cr-chromic chloride intravenously and save the rest for the standard.
3. Arrange for 24 h stools to be collected for 5 days. Supply the ward with:
   (a) five containers and lids
   (b) one container of 40% formaldehyde solution (preservative)
   (c) a copy of the instruction sheet (see Table 11.1)
4. At the end of the 5 day collection, homogenize each sample on a paint can shaker. Before starting to count, ensure that the lids are secured firmly. The containers should be packed in a polythene bag to prevent spills should any of them leak. Count the samples for 5 min each.
5. The standard is prepared by diluting 5 ml of the dose to 1 litre with water. Count the standard under the same conditions as the samples.
6. Background is counted as follows: count a container with 1 litre of water in it.

11.4.4 CALCULATIONS

Calculate the net counts per minute for each sample:

Net counts per minute = Total counts per minute − Background counts per minute

$$\text{Excretion (\%)} = \frac{\text{Net stool counts per minute}}{\text{Net standard counts per minute}} \times 100$$

The normal range is below 1% in the total excretion over 5 days.

11.5 LYMPHATIC IMAGING

11.5.1 PATIENT PREPARATION

Nil.

11.5.2 RADIOPHARMACEUTICAL AND DOSE

35 MBq ^{99}Tc^m-rhenium sulphide colloid

Two syringes with high-specific-activity ^{99}Tc^m-labelled rhenium sulphide colloid, each containing 35 MBq in 0.1 ml, are needed.

11.5.3 PATIENT POSITIONING

The patient is positioned supine on the imaging table with the camera centred over the area to be imaged.

11.5.4 EQUIPMENT

A wide-field-of-view gamma camera fitted with a high-resolution collimator is used.

11.5.5 COMPUTER

If the facility is available, the computer can be used for backing up the study. Record the images using a 128 × 128 word matrix for 5 min per image.

11.5.6 TECHNIQUE

1. The injection site will depend on which lymphatic chain is to be investigated. For example, the patient may be injected subcutaneously in
    (a) the medial two interdigital webs of the foot for studying the leg chain or,
    (b) bilaterally near the manubrium sterni for studying the breast lymphatic chain.
2. As soon as the injections are given, position the patient with the camera centred over the lymphatic chain being investigated, and record images every half-hour for 5 min per view. Occasionally there is rapid transit of the radiopharmaceutical, and this should be monitored carefully using

the persistence scope and the images recorded with shorter intervals.

3. If the injection sites are in the field of view, these should be masked out using appropriate lead shielding. Corresponding ^{57}Co marker images should also be recorded by placing the markers on relative anatomical sites, without moving the patient, so that these can be superimposed on the lymphatic images using the computer. These marker views need only be done for 30 s duration, after peaking the camera on ^{57}Co. Remember to re-peak the camera on ^{99}Tc^{m} setting.

4. Continue imaging until the lymphatic chain is clearly visualized. This may take up to 6 h. It may be helpful to mobilize the patient to increase the lymphatic flow. A cardiac exercise bicycle can be used for this purpose.

INDEX

Abscess
  intra-abdominal 183
  intrahepatic 183
Adrenal cortex imaging 156–7
Adrenal diseases 137
Ankylosing spondylitis 35
Atrial septal defect 99
Avascular necrosis of bone 35

Battered child syndrome (non-accidental injury) 35
Bicycle ergometer exercise procedure 104–6
Biliary (duodenogastric) reflux 58, 70–2
Bone imaging studies 35–44
  bone flow study 42–3
  radiopharmaceuticals 36
  routine 37–8
    using scanning gamma camera 40–1
  sacroiliac quantitation study 44
  whole body positioning 39 (fig.)
Bone marrow imaging 50–1

Calcitonin provocation test 163
Cardiac studies 98–123
  cardiac stress worksheet 115 (table)
  first-pass study for left-to-right shunt detection 118–21
  gated red-cell studies *see* gated red-cell studies
  infarct imaging 110–11
  MAA blood flow study for right-to-left shunt detection 122–3
  myocardial imaging using ^{201}Tl 108–9
  radiopharmaceuticals 100–3
    ^{99}Tc^{m}-labelled HSA microspheres 103
    ^{99}Tc^{m}-pyrophosphate 100
    ^{99}Tc^{m}-RBCs (kit method) 101–2
    ^{201}Tl 100

stannous agent 102–3
stress testing 104–7
  bicycle ergometer exercise procedure 104–6
  Persantin (dipyridamole) stress procedure 106–7
Cardiotoxic drugs, patient taking 99
Cerebral flow studies 128–9
Cisternography 125, 132–3
Coronary artery disease 98
^{51}Cr-labelled chromic chloride 183

Dipyridamole (Persantin) stress procedure 106–7
Duodenogastric (biliary) reflux 58, 70–2

Ejection fraction estimation 99
Endocrine studies 136–63
  adrenal cortex imaging 156–7
  calcitonin provocation test 163
  ^{123}I-perchlorate discharge test 146–7
  phaeochromocytoma imaging using ^{131}I-MIBG 158–9
  radiopharmaceuticals 138–40
    ^{99}Tc^{m}-pertechnetate 138–40
    ^{201}Tl-thallous chloride 140
  testicular imaging 160–1
  thyroid imaging/uptake, using ^{123}I 144–5
  thyroid imaging/uptake/using ^{99}Tc^{m} 141–3
  TRH test 163
  whole-body imaging, using ^{131}I 148–50
Epididymitis 137
Epiphora 183

Frusemide diuresis, two-kidney renal study using 8–9

^{67}Ga citrate 184

^{67}Ga imaging 183, 185–7
  liver-spleen subtraction 187
Gastric (oesophageal) reflux 66–7
Gastric emptying 58
  dual label 68–9
Gastric studies 58–83
  radiopharmaceuticals 60–3
    ^{111}In-labelled fatty drink 61
    ^{111}In-labelled milk drink 62–3
    ^{99}Tc^m-HIDA 60
    ^{99}Tc^m-labelled acidified orange
      drink 60–1
    ^{99}Tc^m-labelled bran in porridge
      61–2
Gastrointestinal blood loss 165
  localization using ^{99}Tc^m-RBCs 78
  study using ^{51}Cr 176–7
Gastrointestinal protein loss estimation,
  using ^{51}Cr-chromic chloride 190–1
Gated red-cell studies 112–17
  procedure for stress gated cardiac
    115–17
  isometric hand grip 116–17
Glomerular filtration rate 27–33
  ^{51}Cr-EDTA dilution/dispensing 28–31
    adult's preparation/procedure 28–9
    child's/infant's preparation/
      procedure 29–31
  ^{51}Cr-EDTA technique 31–3

Haematology studies 164–9
  ^{51}Cr gastrointestinal blood loss 176–7
  plasma volume estimation, using
    ^{125}I-HSA 178–9
  radiopharmaceuticals 166–7
  red-cell mass estimation 168–9
  red-cell sequestration 173–5
  red-cell survival 170–3
Hepatobiliary imaging 64–5
Hydronephrosis, obstructive/
  non-obstructive 1
Hyperparathyroidism 35

Infarct imaging, cardiac 110–11
^{123}I-perchlorate discharge test 146–7
^{123}I sodium iodide 136
^{81}Kr^m gas 86

Lacrimal scintigraphic imaging 188–9
Left-to-right intracardiac shunt 98–9
  first-pass study 118–21

Legg-Perthe's disease 35
Leucocyte imaging, using ^{111}In 180–1
  ^{111}In-leucocyte preparation 183 (fig.)
LeVeen (peritoneal) shunt study 56
Liver
  cold spot 45
  cyst 45
  tumour 45
Liver-spleen studies 45–56
  bone marrow imaging 50–1
  liver-spleen imaging 48–9
  peritoneal (LeVeen) shunt study 56
  radiopharmaceuticals 46–7
  spleen imaging with denatured
    RBCs 52–3
  splenic clearance study 54–5
  subtraction imaging 183, 187
Lung imaging studies 86–97
  ^{81}Kr^m ventilation 92–3
  perfusion 90–1
  radiopharmaceuticals 88–9
  ^{99}Tc^m-DTPA aerosol ventilation 94–5
  ventilation imaging, using ^{133}Xe 96–7
Lymphatic imaging 192–3
Lymphomas 183

Meckel's diverticulum 59
  imaging 76–7
^{131}meta-iodobenzylguanidine 137
Microspheres 86
Myocardial imaging, using ^{201}Tl 108–9
Myocardial infarction, acute 98

Neurological studies 126–35
  cerebral flow studies 128–9
  cisternography 125, 132–3
  radiopharmaceuticals 126–7
  static brain imaging 130–1
  ventriculoatrial shunts 134–5
Non-accidental injury (battered child
  syndrome) 35

Oesophageal clearance 74–5
Oesophageal (gastric) reflux 66–7
Orthoiodohippurate 2
Osteomyelitis 35

Paget's disease 35
Parathyroid imaging 136–7, 151–5
  ^{99}Tc^m injection first 154
  ^{201}Tl injection first 152–3

Peritoneal (LeVeen) shunt 56
Persantin (dipyridamole) stress 106–7
Phaeochromocytoma 137
  imaging, using ^{131}I-MIBG 158–9
Plasma volume 164
  estimation, using ^{125}I-HSA 178–9
Protein leakage into GI tract 183
Pulmonary embolus 86
Pulmonary hypertension 86
Pulmonary inhalation study 59

Renal artery stenosis 2
Red blood cells 164
  ^{51}Cr labelled 164
  mass estimation 168–9
  sequestration 164, 173–5
  survival 164, 170–3
Renal imaging studies 1–25
  radiopharmaceuticals 2–4
    ^{123}I- hippuran 3–4
    ^{99}Tc^m-DMSA 3
    ^{99}Tc^m-DTPA 2–3
Renal transplant study 19–22
Residual bladder volume estimation
  14–15
Right-to-left intracardiac shunt 99
  MAA blood flow study 122–3

Sacroiliac quantitation study 44
Salivary gland imaging
  dynamic 82–4
  static 80–1
Spleen
  clearance study 54–5
  imaging with denatured RBCs 52–3
  see also Liver-spleen studies
Static brain imaging 130–1

Static renal study, using ^{99}Tc^m-DMSA
  23–5
Stress fractures 35

^{99}Tc^m aerosol 87
^{99}Tc^m diethylenetriaminepentaacetic
  acid (DTPA) 1
^{99}Tc^m dimercaptosuccinic acid (SMSA)
  1
^{99}Tc^m methoxyisobutylsonitrile (MIBI)
  98
^{99}Tc^m pertechnetate 58–9, 136
^{99}Tc^m Phyrophosphate (PYP) 98
Testicular imaging 160–1
Testicular torsion 137
Thallium 98
Thyroid diseases 136
Thyroid imaging/uptake, using
  ^{123}I 144–5
  ^{99}Tc^m 141–3
TRH test 162
Two-kidney renal study
  standard dynamic, using ^{99}Tc^m-DTPA
    4–7
  using frusemide diuresis 8–10
  using ^{123}I-hippuran 16–18

Ureteric reflux study 12–13

Ventricular septal defect 99
Ventriculoatrial shunts 134–5
Vesicoureteric reflux 1

White cell imaging, using ^{111}In 164–5
Whole body imaging, using ^{131}I 148–50

^{133}Xe gas 87